The Disease of the Soul

LEPROSY IN MEDIEVAL LITERATURE

The Disease of the Soul

LEPROSY IN MEDIEVAL LITERATURE

Saul Nathaniel Brody

CORNELL UNIVERSITY PRESS

Ithaca and London

Cornell University Press gratefully acknowledges
a grant from the Andrew J. Mellon Foundation
that aided in bringing this book to publication.

First published 1974 by Cornell University Press.
Published in the United Kingdom by Cornell University Press Ltd.,
2-4 Brook Street. London W1Y 1AA.
Second Printing 1975

International Standard Book Number 0-8014-0804-0
Library of Congress Catalog Card Number 73-8407

Printed in the United States of America

For Frohma

man und wîp diu sint al ein;
als diu sunn diu hiute schein,
und ouch der name der heizet tac.
der enwederz sich gescheiden mac:
si blüent ûz eime kerne gar.

Contents

Illustrations

Preface

This book sets out to define and explain a remarkable phenomenon in medieval European literature: the association of leprosy with moral defilement. Of all the diseases that afflicted medieval man, leprosy especially came to be understood as divine punishment for sinfulness and to be viewed as no other sickness known to man has ever been. This is to say neither that leprosy was the only disease coupled with sin nor that such coupling was a medieval invention. Sin and disease were associated from the earliest times, and by the Middle Ages the connection had become traditional. Many writers equated the cardinal sins with particular diseases, for example,[1] and leprosy was only one affliction among many associated with moral perversion; but the notion of leprosy as a moral disease was particularly intense and deeply rooted. Other diseases have lost their medieval connotations, but leprosy has not. Although we no longer think of dropsy as a sinner's disease, much less as

---

[1] See Angus Fletcher, *Allegory: The Theory of a Symbolic Mode* (Ithaca, N.Y., 1964), pp. 199–202; and Morton W. Bloomfield, *The Seven Deadly Sins* (East Lansing, 1952), pp. 8, 28, et passim.

a disease particularly tied to covetousness, leprosy still retains many of its old associations. For instance, the medieval
link between leprosy and lechery still persists. There is no
medical evidence to show that lepers are extraordinarily
lustful, but a venerable tradition insists that they are; and
tradition, not clinical observation, influences this modern
description of leprosy: "Leprosy in its early stages stirs the
venereal appetite in a marked fashion. A strange, unbridled
desire for pleasure flows in the veins of an incipient leper.
One wonders why. . . . The fact is that nobody knows,
not even the doctors. What is certain is that the most phleg-
matic temperaments become curiously sensitive and subject
to the appeal of sex when the disease sets in."[2] It is also tradition which has given us the phrase "moral leper," a commonplace in our language. The idea of leprosy in medieval
literature is not entirely alien to us; although some of the
old ideas have of course vanished, we have preserved the
notion that the disease is always fiercely infectious, and the
disease's tie with immorality is still with us. But because we
have only vague impressions of how the leper was treated
during the Middle Ages we do not fully appreciate the significance of lepers and leprosy in the literature of that time.
For that reason, I attempt here to interpret medieval literature involving leprosy and to evaluate it in the light of its
cultural context.

The documents considered in this study have been selected
because they are pertinent, significant, and representative.
I have not discussed literary works whenever it is doubtful
that they describe lepers,[3] or when dealing with them would

[2] Paolo Zappa, *Unclean! Unclean!*, trans. Edward Storer (London, 1933), pp. 97–98.
[3] One instance is Chaucer's description of the Summoner, who

have been cumbersome and repetitive—as with versions of the widespread Amis and Amiloun story and with many of the instances in which the healing of leprosy through blood appears. Because the number of books and articles on leprosy is awesome, as the volumes of the bibliography on leprosy[4] and the *Index-Catalogue of the Surgeon General's Library* testify, I have chosen critical material only when it appeared particularly relevant and authoritative.

Some comment is necessary here about my method of quoting and offering translations of passages written in foreign languages. For the convenience of nonspecialist readers, I have quoted most of the passages in translation, wherever possible supplying references to texts of the original passages (there are some instances where the only texts available to me were translations). The translations offered are usually mine; where they are not, sources are provided in footnotes. I have quoted passages in the original whenever the sense could not be adequately and accurately conveyed in English prose, as is the case with poetry and literary passages in general. Thus, verse passages are uniformly given in the original, as are prose passages when the language of the original is itself significant, whether because of vocabulary or style.

---

was—so far as I know—first identified as a leper by Walter Clyde Curry, *Chaucer and the Medieval Sciences* (New York, 1926), pp. 37–47. However, it has been shown that the source of Chaucer's description of the Summoner is Vincent of Beauvais' account of the symptoms of scabies, which he differentiates from leprosy. See Pauline Aiken, "The Summoner's Malady," *SP*, XXXIII (1936), 40–44.

[4] *Indice Bibliografico de Lepra*, ed. Luiza Keffer, 3 vols. (São Paulo, 1944–1948).

Finally, it is a pleasure to express my gratitude to those who have given me help during the preparation of this book.

First mention shall be of my wife. My writing of this book must have seemed to her an incurable disease, but she willingly shared my affliction, suffered patiently, and has no doubt had her purgatory on this earth. I dedicate this book to her.

Among the many persons who gave me encouragement while I was writing, four others were especially close to me—my late father, my mother, and my daughters—and by their closeness they made this book possible.

For permission to reproduce illustrations, I am grateful to the Bayerische Staatsbibliothek München, the Bettmann Archive, the Biblioteca Apostolica Vaticana, the Bibliothèque Nationale, the Trustees of the British Museum, the Germanisches Nationalmuseum Nürnberg, the Landesbildstelle Rheinland, and the National Library of Medicine. Specific acknowledgments accompany the plates. Also, I wish to thank the City College Faculty Senate Committee on Research and Publication for a grant which enabled me to obtain the illustrations.

I am indebted to several sources for permission to quote from their works: to Basil Blackwell, Publisher, for *Der Arme Heinrich* and *The Romance of Tristran by Beroul;* to the Council of the Early English Text Society for *Amis and Amiloun;* to Harvard University Press for *Prudentius,* a volume in the Loeb Classical Library series; to Manchester University Press for Robert Henryson's *Testament of Cresseid,* a title in the series Old & Middle English Texts; to the Société des Anciens Textes Français for *Jaufré;* and to Fondation Singer Polignac and Editions A. et J. Picard et Cie for *Oeuvres complètes de Rutebeuf.*

In addition, I wish to thank Cornell University Press for invaluable guidance and assistance while this book was being made ready for publication.

Of those who came to my scholarly assistance, special acknowledgment is due to Rudolph Radna, M.D., of the Department of Health's Tropical Disease Clinic, Washington Heights Center, New York City, for reviewing my discussion of the medical aspects of leprosy; to Professor Walter Dubler, for his assistance in gathering and translating Hebrew commentaries on the Old Testament; to Professor Shalom Paul, for calling to my attention pertinent Old Testament scholarship; to Professor Howard Schless, for his helpful advice and for his painstaking reading and careful criticism of the entire manuscript; to Professor Robert E. Kaske, for his incisive, critical comments; and to Professors E. T. Donaldson, Joan Ferrante, Peter Haidu, and Renata Karlin, who also read the manuscript and helped to improve it.

My deepest obligation is to Professor W. T. H. Jackson of Columbia University, who first suggested this study to me and guided me at every stage in its writing. He made his profound knowledge of medieval literature available to me. I am indebted to him as well for his extraordinary patience, courtesy, and encouragement. I can hardly hope to repay his great kindness.

SAUL NATHANIEL BRODY

New York City

Abbreviations

Arch path Anat Physiol	*Archiv für pathologische Anatomie und Physiologie und für klinische Medicin*
Bull Hist Med	*Bulletin of the History of Medicine*
Bull Soc fr Hist Med	*Bulletin de la Société française d'Histoire de la Médecine*
DVLG	*Deutsche Vierteljahrsschrift für Literaturwissenschaft und Geistesgeschichte*
Edin Med Surg J	*The Edinburgh Medical and Surgical Journal*
EETS, E.S. *or* O.S.	Early English Text Society, Extra Series *or* Original Series
EIC	*Essays in Criticism*
ELN	*English Language Notes*
Gen Prol	General Prologue
Hippocrate	*Hippocrate: Revue d'Humanisme Médicale*
Int J Leprosy	*International Journal of Leprosy*
JAMA	*Journal of the American Medical Association*

J Hist Med	*Journal of the History of Medicine and Allied Sciences*
J Roy Army Med Corps	*Journal of the Royal Army Medical Corps*
Leper Quart	*The Leper Quarterly*
Leprosy Rev	*Leprosy Review*
MA	*Le Moyen Age*
MD Med News	*MD: Medical Newsmagazine*
Med J Rec	*Medical Journal and Record*
MLN	*Modern Language Notes*
MLR	*Modern Language Review*
ParsT	Parson's Tale
PG	*Patrologiae cursus completus: Series graeca*
PL	*Patrologiae cursus completus: Series latina*
PMLA	*Publications of the Modern Language Association of America*
QFSK	*Quellen und Forschungen zur Sprach- und Kulturgeschichte der Germanischen Völker*
SATF	Société des Anciens Textes Français
SP	*Studies in Philology*
ZDA	*Zeitschrift für Deutsches Altertum und Deutsche Literatur*

The Disease of the Soul

LEPROSY IN MEDIEVAL LITERATURE

I

Medical Understandings of Leprosy

> And if he see the leprosy in his skin, and the hair turned white, and the place where the leprosy appears lower than the skin and the rest of the flesh: it is the stroke of leprosy, and upon his judgement he shall be separated.
>
> Leviticus 13:3

This book begins in the twentieth century, for if something is to be said about leprosy in the fiction of the Middle Ages, something must be understood about the disease as it is recognized today. Without a clinical description of it there can be no standard against which to measure the descriptions found in medieval literature. It is intriguing, for example, to discover that the lepers in medieval tales—whether French or German or English—bear remarkably close resemblance to one another and to the medieval textbook cases, but it is unsettling to find that the clinical accounts of the time bear only the most superficial likeness to those written in this century. How can this disparity be explained? The disease has probably altered its form since the Middle Ages, and medieval doctors could not always distinguish leprosy from other skin diseases; at the same time, there is evidence that medieval authors were describing not what they saw but what they thought they ought to see and what their readers expected them to see. Because leprosy presented itself to medieval physicians and writers not merely as a physical but also as a moral disease, they attributed to it signs and symptoms not necessarily or even possibly observable. As the emblem of a moral condition, the disease was not described with modern clinical accuracy, and in order to understand what distortions of its characteristics were involved, we must begin with what a physician of the twentieth century is likely to observe and assume about the disease.

In 1874, Dr. G. H. Armauer Hansen proposed that a bacillus—*Mycobacterium leprae*—is the microbe that causes leprosy. Traditionally, proof for such a theory depends upon the fulfillment of certain conditions first outlined by Robert Koch. In particular, Koch stated that in order to show that a specific organism causes a specific disease, one would first have to isolate the organism in a diseased living being, then grow it outside its host, and finally inoculate and infect a healthy creature with the disease first seen in the original host. Even though no one had been able to apply Koch's postulates to leprosy until 1965, Hansen's proposal was nevertheless universally accepted because of the presence of the organism in all diseased individuals, its absence in healthy ones, and its special effect on body cells.[1]

[1] "Research Barrier Breached: Leprosy Bacillus Grown in Tissue Culture," *JAMA*, CXCII, no. 12 (1965), 32–33, and Charles M. Carpenter and James N. Miller, "The Bacteriology of Leprosy," in *Leprosy in Theory and Practice*, ed. R. G. Cochrane and T. Frank Davy, 2d ed. (Bristol, 1964), p. 13. *Leprosy in Theory and Practice* is cited extensively in this chapter, and referred to simply as "Cochrane." Other medical textbooks and articles are cited only when they differ substantially from Cochrane's book, help explain or amplify information given in it, or supplement it. In general, *Leprosy in Theory and Practice* may be taken as authoritative. In his review of the first edition (ed. R. G. Cochrane

Leprosy is decidedly contagious and is endemic in certain areas of the world. "A reliable estimate of the prevalence of leprosy is impossible from the data available at this time; nevertheless a world total of ten million cases can be accepted."[2] In spite of the wide distribution of the disease, the epidemiology of leprosy appears to present several problems to leprologists, problems concerning its infectiousness and mode of transmission.

Leprosy is variously described as "not essentially different" from other communicable diseases, "less contagious,"[3] "slightly contagious," and "feebly contagious"; but since severe epidemics have been reported in particular areas and since more needs to be known about communicability, it has been recommended that leprosy be called simply "contagious" and that references to the degree of communicability be omitted.[4]

The spread of leprosy seems to depend primarily upon the presence of infectious lepers and their number, and "the risk of infection through contact with these open

[Bristol, 1959]), George L. Fite states, "Certainly this book is better suited to this purpose [of producing a volume for the man who actually treats leprosy] than any of the texts, in any language, of the past. . . . Cochrane has produced the most useful book on leprosy to have been written." See "Book Review: *Leprosy in Theory and Practice*," *Int J Leprosy*, XXVII (1959), 300–302.

[2] *Scientific Meeting on Rehabilitation in Leprosy, Vellore, Madras State, India, 21–29 November, 1960: Report*, World Health Organization Technical Report Series, no. 221 (Geneva, 1961), p. 5. It is understandable that, if an accurate estimate of the numbers of contemporary lepers is extremely difficult to get, no reliable estimates can be given for the Middle Ages.

[3] *Expert Committee on Leprosy: Second Report*, World Health Organization Technical Report Series, no. 189 (Geneva, 1960), p. 25.

[4] L. F. Badger, "Epidemiology," in Cochrane, pp. 75–76.

cases." The risk of infection would appear to be in direct proportion to the intimacy of contact between infected and healthy persons.[5] However, "the natural susceptibility of the host plays an important role in deciding whether or not an individual will develop the disease"—for it has been pointed out on the one hand that most persons are not susceptible to infection, whether through conjugal contact or prolonged contact with leprous patients, and on the other that certain individuals who cannot have had extended, close contact with a leper have developed the disease.[6]

In whatever way a person does become infected, the disease is not likely to reveal itself for some years. The incubation period has not been determined accurately, but the intervals proposed range between three and five years.[7] Ernest Muir states that the period of latency can be from six months to twenty years and that the average period of incubation is about three and one-half years.[8]

The picture of leprosy offered by medieval medicinal tracts departs in significant ways from the contemporary representation. The medieval practitioner never spoke of leprosy as "slightly contagious"; he saw it everywhere. Nor did he find that prolonged, intimate contact with a leper was necessary for the onset of the disease; quite the contrary, he believed it was enough to be downwind from a leper in order to be infected. He had no conception of a long incubation period, for he traced the sources of infection with the confidence with which a food inspector or public health investigator today might attribute an infec-

---

[5] "Epidemiology," pp. 70–73.
[6] *Expert Committee*, p. 4.
[7] "Epidemiology," pp. 73–75.
[8] *Manual of Leprosy* (Baltimore, 1948), pp. 10 f.

tion to rotten meat, or to a particular prostitute. From time to time he might hesitate in making a diagnosis; symptoms *could* be equivocal. Yet if a sufferer showed a particular combination of a limited number of signs, the physician believed that he was confronted with a leper; as he understood it, the forms the disease might take were few and the symptoms fell into simple patterns. The doctor of the Middle Ages viewed one leper as not very different from another, either physically or morally. The contemporary physician does not see so simple a disease. The great disparity between the simplicity of the medieval conception of leprosy and the complexity of the modern one can be demonstrated only by dwelling on detail.

The layman is probably surprised that modern medicine has only very recently succeeded in identifying and distinguishing among the various forms of leprosy. One of the major difficulties faced by leprologists today is the confusion and controversy still surrounding the problem of classification, but in spite of important areas of disagreement, there are certain variant forms of the disease that are universally recognized.[9] The descriptions of leprosy to be given here will stress those forms.

The first indications of leprosy are usually neurological: a patient notices an area of numbness, or feels a sensation of tingling under the skin, or there may be enlargement of certain nerves. Early visible signs may take the form of "alteration in the texture or appearance of the skin, for example, very vague macules."[10] In addition, the patient may

[9] *Expert Committee*, p. 26. See R. G. Cochrane and H. J. Smyly, "Classification," in Cochrane, pp. 299–309.
[10] R. G. Cochrane, "Signs and Symptoms," in Cochrane, p. 252. Unless otherwise noted, descriptions of the signs and symptoms of

suffer slight paralysis of hand muscles, weakening of facial
muscles, and other symptoms due to neurological involvement.[11] Because prognosis is difficult, the first stage of leprosy is called *indeterminate*.[12]

The particular advanced form into which indeterminate
leprosy may develop apparently depends upon the degree
to which body tissues are able to set up an adequate de-
fense against the attacking bacilli.[13] If the tissue response is
effective, the leprosy is said to be *tuberculoid*, a form of the
disease described as benign even though it can deform the
body. If the tissue defenses cannot overcome the bacilli,
lepromatous leprosy—a malignant and progressive variety
—develops. Indeterminate leprosy may become lepromatous,
or the patient may first pass through a *dimorphous* stage[14]
(in which he presents both lepromatous and tuberculoid
symptoms) and then become lepromatous. In general, if a
patient does not receive treatment, the prognosis is grave
with lepromatous leprosy and doubtful with dimorphous
leprosy; in tuberculoid cases, where the tissue response halts
the infection, the prognosis is excellent.[15]

The usually distinctive skin lesions that appear as the
disease progresses are more readily observed than the initial
symptoms and are used in determining whether the leprosy

---

leprosy are taken from this chapter of Cochrane's text, pp. 251–
279.

[11] Chapman H. Binford, "Leprosy," in *Communicable and Infectious Diseases*, ed. Franklin H. Top, 4th ed. (St. Louis, 1960),
pp. 217–219.

[12] V. R. Khanolkar, "Pathology of Leprosy," in Cochrane, p. 126.

[13] R. G. Cochrane, "Classification," pp. 299 ff.

[14] Nomenclature for this phase is confused. Cochrane prefers
dimorphous; others use the terms *borderline* and *intermediate*.

[15] "Classification," pp. 299–309.

is lepromatous, tuberculoid, or dimorphous. In all three
forms, two types of lesions—macular and infiltrated—occur.
Macular lesions are defined as "circumscribed, non-elevated
alterations in the color of the skin of any size or shape."[16]
In lepromatus leprosy, macules are seen in the earlier stages
of the disease; they tend to be scattered symmetrically over
the body, are smooth, shiny, small, and numerous, lack
clear borders between the normal and abnormal skin, and
do not differ in texture from normal skin.

The infiltrated lesions characterize later stages of the
disease. These lesions—in which fluid and cellular elements
have infiltrated the tissue—may take on various appearances. In cases where the infiltrate is diffuse, the skin has a
shiny appearance and the infiltration is difficult to see.
When infiltration is marked, the edges of the lesions become
raised, but the demarcation between normal and affected
skin remains vague. As the disease progresses nodules develop, first on the ears and then anywhere on the surface of
the skin. Ulceration of the nodules may follow, lesions of
the nose and eyes (possibly leading to disfigurement and
blindness) tend to develop, and more or less complete loss
of hair—the disfigurement known as alopecia—may occur.

In contrast to those of the lepromatous form, the macules
of tuberculoid leprosy are large and single or few in number, and they assume asymmetrical distribution. They show
less pigmentation than surrounding skin and are clearly
demarcated from it. The affected area is characterized by
absence of sweating, dryness, scaliness, and often loss of
the ability to sense light touch and heat; in fact, neurological involvement is chacteristic, and in some cases anes-

[16] "Signs and Symptoms," p. 254.

thesia is widespread. Infiltrated lesions in this form of leprosy can be either "minor," with moderate elevation, or "major"— that is, clearly raised and thickened and covering broad areas of the skin.

Dimorphous leprosy is so called because it shows characteristics of both the lepromatous and tuberculoid types. Macular dimorphous leprosy begins with the appearance of one hypopigmented patch, and others gradually develop over the body. While the larger macules have a well-marked edge and show anesthesia, the smaller ones have indistinct borders and no loss of sensation. Infiltrated dimorphous leprosy shows wide distribution of many lesions, often both large and small. Elevation of the lesions occurs at the center and not at the border, which has a vague edge. The skin surface is rough and often scaly, and may or may not show loss of sensation.

During the course of the disease, some lepers develop serious reactions to the presence of the leprosy bacillus in their tissues. In tuberculoid leprosy one lesion may react while others remain unaffected (tuberculoid reaction) or every lesion may show reaction (reactional tuberculoid leprosy). In the first condition some of the more noticeable signs are reddening of the lesions—and in violent reactions, scaling and ulceration of them, accompanied by edema (accumulation of fluid) at the site of the lesions, in the lips, and under the eyelids. In reaction, the lesions become extremely sensitive, and a tapping on them can produce a feeling of burning and pricking. In addition, the feet, hands, and sometimes the nose reveal swelling and tenderness. Reactional tuberculoid leprosy, because it is generalized, produces much greater discomfort: all the lesions are affected, all are tender, and frequently all ulcerate.[17]

In general, the symptoms of reaction in dimorphous leprosy resemble the tuberculoid pattern, except that the course of the reaction is more severe. The leper suffers serious tissue destruction and becomes feeble and emaciated. The lesions become inflamed and then ulcerate acutely, or at the least scale and peel; in this later stage, the leper tends to have a fever which may last for seven months. The nervous system becomes involved, and crippling paralysis and deformation result. When the reaction fades, the leper frequently remains scarred at the sites of the affected lesions—and what is more serious, his disease may change to the lepromatous type.

There are two important types of reaction in lepromatous leprosy. In the first—erythema nodosum leprosum—the nodules of the leper may become elevated and inflamed, producing what are described as "rose spot" nodules; he will experience a fever during the early evening, some possible nerve pain, and other discomfort. Following the reaction, a fair skinned person will have purplish staining at the site of the spots. Scaling of the larger nodules occurs generally. The second kind of reaction in lepromatous leprosy (progressive lepra reaction) begins with general discomfort and develops into a condition marked by small nodules beneath the skin. These may group together and form a hard leathery mass which occasionally ulcerates. Edema of the extremities may occur, and this sometimes produces de-

[17] R. G. Cochrane, "Complicating Conditions Due to Leprosy," in Cochrane, pp. 331–334. All material on reactions is taken from this chapter, pp. 331–343.

formities of the hand or foot. A number of severe complications—particularly of the eye—can accompany this reaction, and if untreated the health of the leper deteriorates:
he becomes increasingly weak and may die of exhaustion
or secondary disorders, such as tuberculosis. Progressive
lepra reaction may last for weeks, months, or even years.
Of all the syndromes of leprosy, the deformity that occurs in advanced cases is perhaps best known and most
often described. The forms that the disfigurement may
take are several.[18] Damage to the nervous system produces
loss of sensation and paralysis of muscles—one manifestation of this is an inability to close the eye, which gives rise
to "a curious unwinking stare";[19] infiltration of the skin
creates puffiness, swelling, wrinkling, and sagging, especially on the face; involvement of tendons may cause par-
tial dislocation of the joints of fingers and toes, or rigidity
of joints; bones—again primarily of the fingers and feet—
may undergo serious deformation, such as collapse of the
joints and shortening of the digits;[20] if cartilage is affected,
finger joints may become stiff and the nose may be ab-
sorbed; and atrophy of the testes may produce alteration of
the secondary sexual characteristics. Lepers who, through
anesthesia, cannot feel pain or heat and cold will suffer
wounds that go unfelt and unnoticed; infection can occur,
and in extreme cases bone marrow or a tendon becomes

[18] See Paul W. Brand, "Deformity in Leprosy," in Cochrane, pp.
447–461.

[19] D. P. Choyce, "The Eyes in Leprosy," in Cochrane, p. 311.

[20] Fingers and toes do not fall off, as is commonly believed.
Rather, the loss of digits is gradual, as in the concentric absorption
of bone caused by decalcification. See D. E. Paterson and C. K.
Job, "Bone Changes and Absorption in Leprosy," in Cochrane,
pp. 425–446.

inflamed, or the leper loses a finger. Those who lose the tactile sense lose the ability to know how hard to hold things, and consequently they place enormous strain on finger tips and tissues; gross deformation of the hand may result. Paralysis or weakening of muscles and nerves can make a person unable to keep his hands and feet in normal position, causing disfigurements such as the "claw hand," clawing of the toes, and foot drop, a condition which forces the leper to walk with a "gait like that of someone about to mount a step."[21] The paralysis may ultimately lead to absorption of fingers. Those who lose the use of certain nerves in the feet become especially prone to chronic ulceration, a condition which often causes entire destruction of the feet.

The alterations that occur in the nose, mouth, and throat are no less hideous.[22] Tuberculoid and dimorphous leprosy produce relatively minor changes in the nose—superficial ulceration and edema and inflammation of the mucous membrane—but alterations in lepromatous leprosy, as usual, are more severe. For instance, chronic inflammation causes erosion of nasal cartilages and bone necrosis; in advanced cases, "extensive nasal involvement presents a tragic picture, with a foul-smelling discharge giving rise to a heavy and musty odour, and with distressing symptoms of nose blockage due to extensive oedema of the mucosa, ulceration, and septic complications with marked crust formations" (p. 324). Involvement of the mouth is similarly more severe in advanced lepromatous cases than in other forms. As the deformation grows extensive, the lips become large, mis-

[21] E. W. Price, "The Care of the Feet," in Cochrane, p. 524.
[22] See Cochrane and Ray P. Breaux, "Lesions of the Nose, Ear, Mouth, and Throat," in Cochrane, pp. 322–330.

shapen, and swollen. The tongue may develop nodules or gross lesions (which may in turn produce deep fissures), and as the process develops, the soft and hard palates and the uvula may also show deformation and mutilation. When the bacilli infect the larynx, the vocal cords may become immobile, causing a characteristic hoarseness in speech, or "harsh whisper" (p. 328). If the condition is ulcerative, the secretions produce not merely hoarseness and pain, but also breathlessness. Whatever the laryngeal involvement, if it develops, the victim may ultimately die of suffocation.

Most persons might expect that leprosy can be diagnosed easily. Since the disfigurements are so gross and horrible, one is likely to suspect that no other condition can possibly resemble it. This simple assumption is far from the truth. Binford writes, "The mimicry of the disease is so great that it has to be differentiated from many diseases, including syphilis, psoriasis, fungous infections, various types of dermatitis, lupus vulgaris, lupus erythematosus, leukoderma, erythema multiforme, peripheral neuritis of other types, Raynaud's disease, and many others."[23] Cochrane has stated, "It is surprising, even in countries where leprosy is endemic, how frequently the disease is misdiagnosed." Furthermore, if leprosy is often diagnosed as another disease, other diseases are often diagnosed as leprosy. Cochrane warns that "the physician who has commenced to take an interest in leprosy is very likely to diagnose everything as leprosy," and he quotes a clinician who remarks that "an individual worker will see only what he is prepared to recognize."[24] The diagnostician, then, can be easily misled

[23] *Communicable and Infectious Diseases*, p. 222.
[24] Cochrane, 1st ed., pp. 143, 154. Cf. J. Ross Innes, "An Approach to the History of Leprosy," *Ciba Symposium*, VII (1959),

not only by the similarity of other diseases to leprosy, but also by his presuppositions, training, and experience—and by his human tendency to find only what he is seeking. Clearly, the obstacles in the way of proper diagnosis are formidable.

They were no less imposing in the Middle Ages. The medieval diagnostician, such as he was, had little available to him in the way of training, textbooks, or sound medical tradition.[25] In all probability, what he brought to the sick bed was what Cochrane and others warn against—a mental set, a bias. Whatever medical manuscripts he might consult were vague enough not to disturb his established notions, and a look at some of those texts will show how stylized and limited they were, and how they contributed to that bias.

One of the greatest limitations in medieval accounts of leprosy is their superficiality. In conducting a physical examination, the modern diagnostician seeks to determine whether lesions are macular or infiltrated, and he observes their size and number, distribution, texture, periphery, and physical sensibility. On the basis of his examination and laboratory tests, he decides whether his patient is suffering

---

118. Innes writes that "accurate knowledge of clinical leprosy is quite common among [primitive peoples]. Where leprosy has been endemic for a long time, the people have a distinct name for it, have a clear clinical picture in their minds of its several manifestations, and can diagnose it with precision. Only where the endemic is recent in its rise is there much confusion with other diseases." Nonetheless, he points out that what was called leprosy in the Middle Ages "included many peeling or scabby or scaling diseases" (pp. 118 f.).

[25] The diagnosis of lepers in the Middle Ages was not performed by doctors only. The clergy, civil officers, juries of citizens, and even lepers were also given the responsibility. See Chapter II.

from indeterminate, dimorphous, tuberculoid, lepromatous, or some other variant of leprosy. The medieval physician was unaware of such subtleties. His descriptions of skin lesions are rarely more specific than "a horrible state of skin with blotches and eruptions" or "hard, stony eminences are felt, on account of the cold black bile." In his concentration upon the obvious and the horrible, he did not usually make fine distinctions, and his descriptions of leprosy are often disorganized, meandering, cursory lists of signs.

Although at the purely empirical level the physician could produce an accurate observation, when theory came into play, tradition would take over and shape what was observed. The evidence of personal experience could be subordinated to conventional notions and procedures, or shaped by them. An instance will suggest one way in which accuracy could be confounded by theory.

When Theodoric of Cervia (1205–1298) discusses leprosy he discriminates something that few other physicians, whether medieval or modern, are likely to observe—the phase of indeterminate leprosy: "Now the signs of incipient lepra are as follows: a common sign at the beginning of all lepra is that spots appear and quickly disappear. Likewise a common sign is the insensibility of certain areas."[26] Cochrane is able to say little more than Theodoric about the symptoms. In the first edition of his text, he reports what "a careful questioning of patients who belong to the white races" suggests: "Such areas of anesthesia may re-

[26] "Lepra" (book III, chap. 55), *The Surgery of Theodoric* (1266), trans. Eldridge Campbell and James Colton, II (New York, 1960), 168. Further references to this work give page numbers of the second volume in parentheses.

main or extend, and later on visible skin lesions may appear. Workers, however, who have studied them have shown that, as a group, these early lesions of leprosy have a great tendency to self-healing, and this probably takes place in a considerable portion of cases, more particularly in children."[27] Theodoric's observation of the transient lesions and numbness, then, apparently has a firm basis in fact, but the conclusions he draws from the examination of blood have no basis at all.

Theodoric states that if three grains of salt dissolve immediately in a patient's blood, this constitutes a sign of incipient leprosy. Another sign is if blood squeaks or is greasy when rubbed in the palm (p. 168). Theodoric surely did not observe any coincidence between these signs and leprosy, though since he apparently expected to find the correlation, he may have persuaded himself of it. This capacity for combining fact and fantasy is typical of medieval medicine. Another writer may challenge the salt test—"and of [the statement] that salt sprinkled over the blood if it melt they are leprous if not they are healthy and contrariwise; it is all false"—but still go on to accept other ideas equally without empirical substantiation: "The limbs tremble and they suffer from irregular pulsation of the heart as if afflicted with heart disease. Those who have been infected by lying with a woman with whom a leper has lain feel this at once."[28]

The humoral theory was one of the common assumptions that subverted clinical observation. The theory presupposes

[27] "Signs and Symptoms," p. 121.
[28] "A Thirteenth Century Clinical Description of Leprosy," ed. and trans. Charles Singer, *J Hist Med*, IV (1949), 238. The Latin text is given on pp. 238–239.

that the world is composed of four elements: fire, air, water, and earth. Each of the elements is linked with one of the four principal body fluids (the cardinal humors), and each of the fluids thereby assumes certain qualities of the elements. Thus, since fire is hot and dry, and since fire is linked with yellow bile (choler), yellow bile is hot and dry. Air is associated with blood, and blood is therefore hot and moist; water is the element of phlegm, the humor which is moist and cold; and earth is the element of the melancholic humor, back bile, which is cold and dry.[29] Moreover, each humor is associated with a color, a taste, an age, a season of the year, and a temperament. For instance, blood has a ruddy color, is bitter, rules in maturity, abounds in spring, and causes wildness of spirit.

The proper balance of humors characterizes health, whereas any imbalance, whether an excess or a deficiency of a humor, causes an alteration of the normal condition. A man in whom blood predominates is "benevolent, jolly, simple, moderate, bland, and sleepy, or fat"; he is sanguine. An overabundance of blood produces "alienation of the mind, as evidenced by laughter and singing."[30] Clearly, the humoral theory was attractive because it explained a man's condition methodically, fully, and in a way consistent with the underlying assumption of a world of four elements.

Theodoric, along with most other physicians of his time, accepts the humoral theory and finds in consequence that there are four kinds of leprosy: "And according to the

[29] Cecelia C. Mettler, *History of Medicine*, ed. Fred A. Mettler (Philadelphia, 1947), p. 9.
[30] David Riesman, *The Story of Medicine in the Middle Ages* (New York, 1935), pp. 304–306.

ancients there are four types of lepra: elephantic, which has to be produced from black bile infecting the blood; leonine, from bile corrupting the blood; tyrian from phlegm infecting the blood; alopecian from corrupt blood" (p. 168).

Since blood is linked with the hot and moist element, air, Theodoric finds that in alopecian leprosy the face is swollen and puffy: "the eyes water; the veins about the eyes and in the face puff up; the nostrils are stuffed up; the gums putrefy and puff up"; "excessive dampness covers the whole body." Furthermore, since alopecian leprosy is associated with blood and the color red, the color of the face is "reddish verging to earthy color and the like" and "the body is marked with reddish spots." (Leonine leprosy, on the other hand, caused by yellow bile, is detectable by "yellowishness of the face verging on the reddish; yellowish color over the whole body.") Sanies—bloody matter— flows from the gums; "with slight palpation of the nostrils blood issues forth"; "the urine is reddish"; "the blood drawn from a vein appears thick and viscous"; in general, "a sanguinary constitution of the body is evident" (pp. 169, 170).

Could Theodoric ever have seen a patient with this combination of signs? It is possible but very unlikely. To be sure, certain forms of leprosy are marked by some of the signs he records, and other diseases may be characterized by others of them. But Theodoric's description is based upon theory, not practice; he seems to have combined signs that would appear together if leprosy were in fact caused by an excess of the sanguinary humor. In brief, Theodoric's work suggests how the medieval physician was subject to tradition, how he could at one moment produce an accurate observation and at the next set aside the evidence of his senses because prevailing theory could not accommodate it.

At the same time, Theodoric seems aware of the disparity between theory and practice, for he warns his readers that the clinical presentations of leprosy will not necessarily fit solely into one of the four categories: "Yet it happens very rarely that it arises from a single humor. Rather more frequently it arises from two or three or four intermingling their parts, from which there appear different and composite signs which can be comprehended by their components" (p. 168). He appends "the general signs of lepra" (pp. 170–171) to his description of the humoral types of leprosy, perhaps in order to provide a summary of the disease, but perhaps also to present a description free from the categories of the humors. Seven of those twelve general, or common, signs are matched by signs recorded by modern leprologists. For instance, Theodoric states that the hair falls from the body, particularly the face, where the eyelashes and eyebrows are lost; this depilation corresponds to the leprous alopecia of nodular lepromatous leprosy and to an ocular involvement common in lepromatous leprosy.[31] According to Theodoric, it is a common sign of leprosy that the eyes themselves become round (previously, he limited this condition to elephantia and leonine leprosy) and the whites livid. The roundness may be the "curious, unwinking stare" of lepromatous leprosy (p. 311), and the lividness of eyes does occur in leprosy. The constriction of nostrils which Theodoric mentions, and the resultant nasal

[31] Cochrane, pp. 266, 310. Further page references to Cochrane are given in parentheses in the following paragraphs.

speech and snoring, are typical signs in tuberculoid, dimorphous, and lepromatous leprosy (pp. 323–324). Involvement of the throat in advanced lepromatous leprosy (p. 325) seems also to have been observed by Theodoric, who affirms that "the voice wavers, tending to lower, or to thinness, from which it finally grows hoarse and the voice fails completely." Furthermore, he takes note of the characteristic anesthesia, though for some reason he lists insensibility of the ankle bone and leg only. Finally, Theodoric states that the face of the leper is ruddy, and tends toward a darker color. Hyperpigmentation occurs in leprosy, and Theodoric's observation of the range of color variation is reliable (although it is not consistent with his description of leonine leprosy, in which he remarks that one of the signs is "yellowness of the face verging on the reddish"; accordingly, the range would have to be from yellow to darker, not ruddy to darker).

Nevertheless, in spite of the correspondence between Theodoric's observations and those of modern physicians, his picture of the disease is still faulty. He presents only seven signs that correspond with signs seen in leprosy; the seven do not necessarily occur simultaneously; and most of them are seen in other diseases. In short, his description could help a doctor diagnose leprosy, but it is too brief to be an adequate guide; moreover, because Theodoric's description also includes signs not seen in leprosy and signs which are too vaguely described, it is as likely to mislead the doctor as to properly aid him.

For example, where Theodoric reports that "the soft parts of the ear are shrunken," Cochrane states that in lepromatous leprosy "the ear lobes are usually appreciably thickened" (p. 263); Cochrane's text makes no mention of "changing color of the nails, with spurts of clear blood if the nail is compressed"; Theodoric states the leprosy is characterized by "corrupt sweating," but Cochrane's book makes no reference to such a phenomenon. Theodoric apparently distinguishes between "nodules" and "hard, stony eminences." Because his treatment of leprous lesions is not detailed, precisely what he means to suggest is not clear. His terms very probably describe several kinds of aggravated skin conditions, but there is the possibility that he is distinguishing between the "succulent" nodules of infiltrated lepromatous leprosy and the "whipcord-like feel of the tuberculoid lesions" (p. 265). The statement that "the face becomes puffy" is unfortunately as vague as his description of the lesions. Indeed, some forms of leprosy do render the face puffy, but the adjective is hardly capable of accounting for the variety of changes in facial appearance which leprosy can cause. Finally, his observation that the blood of lepers "appears harsh and sour" is not confirmed by Cochrane's text.

Theodoric omits from his list of the general signs of leprosy certain conditions that he describes in distinguishing among the varieties of leprosy linked with the humors. Some of the omitted symptoms—such as deformations of the lips and tongue—are frequent and obvious in advanced lepromatous cases, whereas others—observations on the condensation of blood, for example—are fanciful. In any case, of the general signs he *does* present, almost half either do not correspond to conditions recognized by modern leprologists or are too vague to assist in diagnosis. Theodoric's description of leprosy, by reason of its cursoriness and unreliability, could lead a doctor to suspect any aggravated skin condition of being leprosy.

In general, other medieval medical treatises are as undependable as Theodoric's: descriptions of leprosy usually are pictures of combinations of leprosy and other diseases. The explanation for the frequent unreliability of medieval medical accounts is clearly the rudimentary level of medical knowledge in the Middle Ages. Physicians were unskilled and untrained, and their theories were usually faulty; they could not help but be unreliable. Medieval doctors could not properly describe leprosy because they could not tell it apart from scabies, psoriasis, eczema, and a host of other skin conditions. For instance, Charles Singer's examination of a thirteenth century description of leprosy leads him to conclude, "Doubtless it embraces a whole series of pathological states." The inability of medieval physicians to distinguish among diseases was common. Singer writes:

Medieval medical literature is extremely poor in clinical descriptions. Disease entities, as we know them, were hardly recognized. They could scarcely be classified under the then prevalent doctrine—that the body was made up of "four humours," an excess or defect of one or more of which produced symptoms. A few conditions, such as quartan or tertian fever, have constant and unmistakable symptoms and the medieval designations of these are definite and reliable enough. But most of the medieval terms for the diseases, such as "scrofula," "putrid fever," "iliac passion," etc., cover a wide variety of conditions. This was eminently true of "leprosy."[32]

[32] "A Thirteenth Century Clinical Description," p. 237. See also George Newman, "On the History of the Decline and Final Extinction of Leprosy as an Endemic Disease in the British Islands," *Prize Essays on Leprosy*, The New Sydenham Society, CLVII (London, 1895), p. 5: "There can, I think, be no doubt that many and various diseases were included in the comprehensive term 'leprosy.'"

Typically, then, descriptions of leprosy are gathered from "a whole series of pathological states," including true leprosy. We might expect the lists of signs and symptoms to be excessively complicated and numerous in consequence; instead, we find relatively brief lists, relatively simple descriptions. The number of signs rarely exceeds twenty or thirty, yet a careful picture of true leprosy alone could easily present twice thirty signs.[33]

The relative brevity of medieval descriptions of leprosy is determined partly by the contexts in which most of them appear. Usually, medical treatises of the time are encyclopedic; they attempt to discuss all the known diseases (Theodoric's *Surgery* is divided into four books; the chapter on leprosy is the fifty-fifth of the third book). In writing such a work, the author must necessarily be as concise as possible.

Under the best circumstances, brevity in medical writing can be achieved only at the expense of thoroughness, and consequently a medical description in an encyclopedia of diseases will necessarily be incomplete. Whether or not it will be accurate depends upon the resources available to the author and upon the breadth of his experience.

Clearly, medieval encyclopedic texts were predisposed to be inexact, since the medical writer had little sound information available to him and his experience with the diseases he wrote about was necessarily limited. Most physicians of any age never encounter *all* the illnesses they

[33] In summarizing the characteristic physical features of macules, Cochrane gives fifteen special attributes—five each for tuberculoid, lepromatous, and dimorphous leprosy. In discriminating infiltrated lesions of tuberculoid and dimorphous leprosy, he cites twelve—six for tuberculoid and six for dimorphous leprosy. (See "Signs and Symptoms," pp. 258, 268.) Thus, in two tables which briefly and partially summarize the appearance of *lesions only*, Cochrane lists twenty-seven signs.

study in medical school, and some of those they do see are seen very rarely. In consequence, modern medicine has witnessed the rise of specialists, a phenomenon attested to by Cochrane's *Leprosy in Theory and Practice.* The book, a study of one disease, has thirty-three chapters and seven appendixes written by forty-three contributors.

Specialists were unknown in the Middle Ages. If a medical writer had any pretentions, they were to expertness in all illnesses rather than to specialization in one. Thus, in writing a treatise on diseases, he wrote as briefly as possible about many illnesses that he knew very little about. It naturally became a major problem for him to appear learned and experienced where he was not.

He could achieve the appearance of wisdom by calling upon the authority of tradition, citing authorities, and copying from authorities without citing them. The reverence for medical authorities is reflected in Chaucer's description of the doctor who rides among the Canterbury pilgrims. When Chaucer (ca. 1343–1400) wants to suggest the excellence of his physician, he catalogues the medical sages known by him:

> Well knew he the olde Esculapius,
> And Deyscorides, and eek Rufus,
> Olde Ypocras, Haly, and Galyen,
> Serapion, Razis, and Avycen,
> Averrois, Damascien, and Constantyn,
> Bernard, and Gatesden, and Gilbertyn.[34]

[34] Gen Prol, ll. 429–434, in *The Works of Geoffrey Chaucer,* ed. Fred N. Robinson, 2d ed. (Boston, 1957). Muriel Bowden observes, "All the medical authorities of antiquity are here . . . and Chaucer has not omitted the important men of his own nation." See *A Commentary on the General Prologue to The Canterbury Tales* (New York, 1948), pp. 200–202.

The medieval veneration of authority is seen directly in a formulary written by one of Chaucer's contemporaries, Johannes de Mirfeld (d. 1407). Johannes, in assembling a prescription book for laymen, does not claim to have put together an original collection. Rather, in order to make his work authoritative, he denies any originality and "confines himself to copying wholesale from the standard medical books of his day. To produce a full list of his sources would involve writing a bibliography of practically the whole of medieval medical literature."[35] The indiscriminate borrowing that characterizes medieval medical writing had the sanction of generations of practice. Arabic treatises are based upon works attributed to Hippocrates (460–377 B.C.) and upon commentaries on them by Galen (130–ca. 200). The Arabic writers "seem to have never entirely abandoned the notion that they were but humble disciples following in the footsteps of great masters, whom they were bound to revere, imitate, and quote, but never overthrow." Their attitude was adopted by their heirs, medieval physicians who plagiarized medical textbooks by stringing together excerpts copied from authorities, without regard for confirming the truth of the statements.[36]

Medieval descriptions of leprosy, with their remarkable similarity, demonstate the way in which medical writers followed tradition and one another. A medical historian, Hans Carlowitz, has made a point of comparing most of the important thirteenth and fourteenth century writers on leprosy: Gilbertus Anglicus (fl. 1245), Theodoric, William

[35] Percival Horton-Smith Hartley and Harold Richard Aldridge, *Johannes de Mirfeld of St. Bartholomew's, Smithfield: His Life and Works* (Cambridge, Eng., 1936), p. 41.

[36] Hartley and Aldridge, p. 42.

of Saliceto (1210–1280), Lanfranc (d. ca. 1306), Arnald of
Villanova (ca. 1235–1311), Bernard Gordon (ca. 1260–
1308), Henry of Mondeville (ca. 1260–1320), Vital du
Four (d. 1327), John of Gaddesden (1280?–1361), and
Guy of Chauliac (ca. 1300–1368). He observes that the
authors differ from one another only slightly and that all
those who lived after Bernard made use of his *Lilium medicinae* (1303). He notes that Henry of Mondeville and John
of Gaddesden are particularly alike; they frequently use
the same phraseology, for example. Carlowitz concludes
that all the named authors relied less upon their own observations than upon the work of the famous Arabian physicians—Rhazes (850–923), Haly Abbas (d. 994), Avicenna
(980–1037), and so forth—and their eleventh century com-
mentator, Constantinus Africanus (ca. 1020–1087); in addition, he confirms the observation of Hartley and Aldridge
that, for their own part, the Arabians borrowed heavily
from Greek sources.[37]

The medieval reverence for authority and tradition, and
the profound effect it had on medical literature, can hardly
be overemphasized. The pronouncements of the ancients
were passed on from writer to writer, and much that was
valuable was preserved in this way, but just as often the
transmitted information was faulty, confused, or fanciful.
Tradition, maintained through copying, kept inaccuracies
as well as accuracies alive, even in those authors who most
clearly distrusted tradition.

For example, Guy of Chauliac shows his suspicion of
the humoral theory by dividing his description of leprosy

[37] [Constantin] Hans Carlowitz, ed., *Der Lepraabschnitt aus
Bernhard von Gordons "Lilium medicinae" in mittelalterlicher
deutscher Uebersetzung* (Leipzig, 1913), p. 9.

into unequivocal and equivocal signs—signs that he believed always signify leprosy and those that are seen not only in leprosy but in other diseases as well.[38] Guy's approach is thus remarkably empirical, but his list includes signs that are unobservable; significantly, several of them are similar to those given by other medieval authors. As an instance, both Theodoric and Guy advise that the color of urine should be examined as a diagnostic test; the procedure has no validity. Similarly, both doctors agree that a leper's blood may be of a special character. Guy reports that lepers may have black, livid, dark blood which is ashy, gritty and clotted. According to Theodoric, in elephantia the color of the blood is earthen and ashen, and the blood "condenses" (clots) quickly; alopecian blood is thick and viscous, and it grows dark and sticky when washed.

A scrutiny of Guy's list of signs and symptoms proves him to be cursory in the typical fashion of medieval medical writers—syndromes are pat and easily defined. Although he may be more the empiricist than Theodoric, Guy too observes the unobservable. We cannot be sure why—he may have convinced himself that indeed he saw what in truth was not there, or it may be that he was satisfying his readers, who required him to say something about blood and urine. There is little doubt a doctor's patients expected it of him; in fact, they often tested his ability. (Incidents of this kind occurred so frequently that Arnald of Villanova instructed physicians on how to guard themselves against patients who tricked their doctors when submitting urine samples for examination.[39]) However it was—whether

[38] See "De Ladrerie," in *La Grande Chirvrgie* (1363), ed. E. Nicaise (Paris, 1890), pp. 401–412.

[39] Henry E. Sigerist, "Bedside Manners in the Middle Ages: The Treatise *De Cautelis Medicorum,* Attributed to Arnald of

because of Guy's bias or his patients'—the tradition is pre-served; the overall effect of Guy's text is to present a sim-plified view of leprosy and to perpetuate misconceptions.

The medieval tendency to follow tradition is represented widely. Latin poets of the classical period regularly bor-rowed from Greek poets and from one another, and this same readiness to borrow is seen in later Christian writers.[40] Medieval artists similarly copy from one another or fit new shapes to familiar outlines and patterns. For example, an illustration of a lion by Villard de Honnecourt (fl. 1230–1235) is highly stylized ("it looks like an ornamental or heraldic image"), but Villard states that he drew the animal from life. E. H. Gombrich comments, "He can have meant only that he had drawn his schema in the presence of a real lion. How much of his visual observation he allowed to enter into the formula is a different matter." A comparable instance of an artist's rendering the unfamiliar in terms of the familiar is seen in representations of the human body by Leonardo da Vinci (1452–1519): "The greatest of all the visual explorers, Leonardo himself, has been shown to have made mistakes in his anatomical drawings. Apparently he drew features of the human heart which Galen made him expect but which he cannot have seen."[41] Similarly, in manu-

---

Villanova," in *Henry E. Sigerist on the History of Medicine*, ed. Felix Marti-Ibañez (New York, 1960), pp. 131–132.

[40] Henry Osborn Taylor, *The Classical Heritage of the Middle Ages* (New York, 1958), pp. 291–292. Ernst Robert Curtius re-marks that it is "the case with almost all medieval citations" that they are quoted without mention of their sources. See *European Literature and the Latin Middle Ages*, trans. Willard R. Trask (New York, 1963), p. 28.

[41] *Art and Illusion: A Study in the Psychology of Pictorial Representation* (New York, 1960), pp. 78–79, 83.

script illuminations and early woodcuts, lepers are con-
ventionally represented with numerous spots, small circles,
or other marks intended to depict lesions on their bodies.
There is little attention to anatomical accuracy, for the
artist has as his overriding purpose to give the viewer a
symbol that can be immediately understood; he draws the
leper according to the traditional symbolic pattern rather
than from life. Illuminations of Job from the twelfth and
fourteenth centuries show him with a spotted body, just
as a woodcut from the early sixteenth century does (figs.
1–3). Naaman the leper is similarly shown covered with
spots (fig. 4). Three illuminations of Jesus curing leprosy
also show spotted lepers, and in each illumination Jesus extends his right hand toward the lepers, who all approach
with arms extended, as if in supplication (figs. 5–7). An
illumination of Aaron performing the function assigned
him by Moses in Leviticus 13 follows the same pattern as
the representations of Jesus and lepers, possibly because
Aaron was understood as prefiguring Jesus; his head is surrounded by a nimbus, he wears vestments similar to Jesus',
and he extends his right hand toward a supplicating leper
(fig. 8). In each of the representations, even in those that
seem most attentive to accurate portrayal of lepers' costumes (figs. 9 and 10), the artist does not imitate the physical appearance of living lepers but reproduces the emblem
of leprosy—a body covered with spots.[42]

[42] See also Eugen Holländer, *Die Medezin in der klassischen
Malerei*, 3d ed. (Stuttgart, 1923), pp. 153 ff. (figs. 90 ff.); and
Gertrud Schiller, *Ikonographie der christlichen Kunst*, I (Gütersloh, 1966), 183–184, 462–463 (figs. 530–535). Holländer and Schiller
show spotted lepers in a variety of media, including illumination,
fresco, embossed metal, and ivory.

Medical writers clearly follow tradition in the way the artists do; like the artists, they copy from one another and produce descriptions of leprosy that conform to description in their sources. Moreover, the medical accounts seem to have influenced portrayals of lepers in medieval literature. Literary lepers are very much like lepers in medical treatises: the faces of both types are covered with nodules, their breath stinks, and they speak with altered (and usually hoarse) voices. A striking example of such a leper is Cresseid in Robert Henryson's *Testament of Cresseid*, a fifteenth-century poem.[43] Cresseid is described with great exactness,[44] and the signs of her leprosy are those cited by the medieval physicians. It may be that what Henryson selected from personal observation to include in his description was determined by what the medieval physicians made him expect to see. It is also possible that he modeled his description directly after one in a medical treatise,[45] just as Chaucer did in his depiction of the Summoner.[46] In any event, that Henryson's description was shaped more

[43] Ed. Denton Fox (London, 1968). The quotation from the poem that appears below is followed by line numbers in brackets.

[44] The exactness of Henryson's description has led some mistakenly to suppose that since he reports the same symptoms as the medical writers, he must have based his description on firsthand observation of lepers. See Marshall W. Stearns, *Robert Henryson* (New York, 1949), pp. 44–45; and the source he cites, J. Y. Simpson, "Antiquarian Notices of Leprosy and Leper Hospitals in Scotland and England, Part II," *Edin Med Surg J*, LVII (1842), 139–140.

[45] This suggestion, which Stearns takes note of, is made by Johnstone Parr, "Cresseid's Leprosy Again," *MLN*, LX (1945), 487–491. See also Fox, pp. 25–26.

[46] Pauline Aiken, "The Summoner's Malady," *SP*, XXXIII (1936), 40–44.

by tradition than by empirical observation is confirmed by the "spottis black" (349) that mar Cresseid's complexion. Such spots are not characteristic of true leprosy,[47] although they are among the signs described by the medieval physicians. For example, Bartholomaeus Anglicus (fl. 1225) mentions diverse specks in four colors—either red, black, wan, or pale[48]—possibly corresponding to the four humors. There is in any case no doubt that Cresseid's spots are a sign that her leprosy is melancholic in origin.[49] When Saturn (who himself has a melancholic complexion and who has jurisdiction over leprosy) stands over Cresseid and announces her sentence, he says:

> I change thy mirth into melancholy,
> Quhilk is the mother of all pensiuenes;
> Thy moisture and thy heit in cald and dry.
>   [316–318]

But Cresseid's spots conform not only to what the traditional humoral theory requires. They are also distinctive of lepers in medieval manuscript illuminations; to be sure, they

[47] Beryl Rowland, "The 'seiknes incurabill' in Henryson's *Testament of Cresseid*," *ELN*, I (1963–64), 176, points out that the spots are not even a sign of syphilis—the disease which, she argues, Henryson describes.

[48] *De Proprietatibus Rerum* (ca. 1266), trans. John Trevisa (London, 1535), book VII, chap. lxv. The passage is quoted in Fox's edition of the *Testament*, p. 25.

[49] Marshall W. Stearns, "Robert Henryson and the Leper Cresseid," *MLN*, LIX (1944), 265–269. Fox points out (p. 33) that Cresseid's black spots are matched by the black spots that are an attribute of Cynthia, the moon (see l. 260), who is, according to astrological traditions, "definitely connected in some way with the leprous infection" (Johnstone Parr, "Cresseid's Leprosy Again," p. 488).

are the essential characteristic in emblematic drawings of lepers. Henryson's demonstrable reliance upon convention is not exceptional; in general, medieval representations of lepers—whether in manuscript illuminations, medical treatises, or poetry—conform to traditional patterns.

The force of tradition in shaping and perpetuating medical misapprehensions about leprosy is seen clearly in the medieval discussions of the causes of leprosy and the moral depravity of lepers. Since ancient times, leprosy has been considered an unclean disease, and its victims have long been linked with moral impurity. Tradition transmitted by copying helped perpetuate the idea of a leper as an emblem of spiritual corruption—and the moral associations of leprosy surround the disease during the Middle Ages.

Medieval medical authors frequently list psychological conditions among the signs that characterize leprosy. Theodoric writes the lepers "grow angry very easily, and more easily than was customary. Evil, crafty habits appear; patients suspect everyone of wanting to hurt them" (p. 171). The thirteenth century description edited by Singer gives the following signs: "horrible dreams . . . bad habits of life . . . They are afraid in sleep. . . . Many burn with desire for coitus. . . . They gladly have intercourse with the healthy but if a healthy person who is also unacquainted with their ailment, as, for example, children, looks on them in the face they are afraid, their faces are troubled, and they despair even for that."[50] Guy of Chauliac states that lepers are "schemers and deceivers, they are furious, and they wish to impose themselves upon the people . . . they have heavy and grievous dreams." Therefore, the diagnostician

[50] "A Thirteenth Century Clinical Description," pp. 237–238.

should ask lepers and their acquaintances "about their craftiness and morals, about their dreams and desires."[51]

The medical writers are generally agreed that lepers threaten society not only through infection but also through their corrupt and evil behavior. Nearly always they specify —and thereby warn—that lepers burn with desire for sexual intercourse. To be sure, most writers describe leprosy itself as a venereal disease.[52]

[51] *La Grande Chirvrgie*, pp. 404, 405. Further instances of medical descriptions of lepers' malice and vices are cited by Ernest Wickersheimer, "Les Accusations d'empoisonnement portées pendant la première moitié du XIVe siècle contre les lépreux et les juifs; leurs relations avec les épidémies de peste," *Comptes-rendus du quatrième congrès international d'histoire de la médecine*, ed. Tricot-Royer and Laignel-Lavastine (Anvers, 1927), pp. 81–82.

[52] The view of leprosy as venereal and of lepers as sexually inflamed no doubt had some basis in fact. They might call any disfiguring skin condition leprosy, and there seems to be little question that venereal diseases were so identified. Further, considering that lepers in asylums were sexually segregated and thereby prevented from having normal sexual relations, it might well appear that they evinced unnatural sexual drives. It has been pointed out that prostitutes were sometimes brought into asylums (Pierre Jonin, *Les Personnages féminins dans les romans français de Tristan au XIIe siècle: Étude des influences contemporaines*, Publication des annales de la faculté des lettres, Aix-en-Provence, new series, no. 22 [Gap, 1958], p. 113) and the leper houses consequently were forced to forbid the entry of "women of light fame and evil reputation," as the house at St. Albans put it (James Y. Simpson, "Antiquarian Notices of Leprosy and Leper Hospitals in Scotland and England, Part I," *Edin Med Surg J*, LVI [1841], 315–316). On the other hand, the common physical condition of the medieval leper—whatever his actual disease—was probably severe enough to weaken him significantly. In all likelihood, he rapidly lost his sexual desire along with his health, and even if he did not entirely lose his sexual drive, neither did he feel it to be heightened. The idea that his sexuality was enhanced by his disease was a myth of

Francis Adams, in his survey of the writings of early Greek, Latin, and Arabian writers,[53] shows that the earliest Greek and Latin writers distinguish, for the most part, between elephantiasis (that is, elephantia) and leprosy, but that Arabian texts tend to view elephantia as a type of leprosy. Among many of the authors he cites there is agreement that both diseases are contagious. At any rate, medieval texts generally seem to follow Albucasis (936–1013) in classifying elephantia as one of the four humoral varieties of leprosy.

The connection of elephantia with sexual intercourse is found in the writing of Aretaeus (second century A.D.), who describes the symptoms of the disease and explains that it is sometimes called satyriasis, "from the redness of the cheeks, and the irresistable and shameless impulse *ad coitum*."[54] Aëtius (fl. 550) states that elephantia is marked by strong venereal desires, and like Aretaeus he observes that it can be spread through contagion.[55] A Sanskrit work of about A.D. 400, the *Ayurvedas* by Susruta, characterizes elephantia as a punishment for unchastity and a sign of sin which can be traced back "to the dreadful nocturnal mysteries of the wife of Brahma, and its shameful commerce. Copulation, contact of the body . . . the same bed . . . such are the causes which convey these dreadful diseases to others."[56] Albucasis describes leprosy as a highly con-

---

the sort that commonly attaches to sinners. In our time, for example, it is commonly assumed that narcotics addicts burn with sexual desire; in truth, they lose it.

[53] *The Seven Books of Paulus Aegineta*, II (London, 1846), 1–15.

[54] *The Extant Works of Aretaeus, the Cappadocian*, ed. and trans. Francis Adams (London, 1856), p. 368.

[55] *Paulus Aegineta*, II, 9, 10.

[56] Summarized in J. R. Whitwell, *Syphilis in Earlier Days* (Lon-

tagious and hereditary disease; Rogerius' description (ca. 1170) parallels Albucasis' and adds that leprosy is contracted by coitus. John of Gaddesden warns that a man who sleeps with a woman who has previously had intercourse with a leper will contract the disease. Bernard Gordon adds that the man will become leprous only if the woman still retains the seminal fluid of the leper. He provides the case of a medical bachelor who contracted the disease through intercourse with a certain lady suffering from leprosy.[57] Robert Copland's English translation of Guy advises the diagnostician "to enquyre yf he hath had the company of any lepresse woman. And yf any lazare had medled with her afore hym and lately bycause of the infect mater and contagyous fylth that she hadde receyved of hym."[58] Theodoric writes, "A person becomes infected, also, from coitus with anyone suffering from lepra, sometimes after coitus calidi and sometimes after coitus frigidi" (p. 178). Almenar, at the beginning of the sixteenth century (1502), teaches that kissing and sexual intercourse can result in a

---

don, 1940), pp. 25–27. It has been suggested that Susruta's text follows Greek medicine as transmitted by the Arabians. In any case, the *Ayurvedas* was known to one Arabian physician by about A.D. 932. See H. Julius Eggeling, "Sanskrit," *Encyclopedia Britannica*, 11th ed., XXIV (New York, 1911), 182 b. The availability to the West not merely of the Indian text but more importantly of the tradition is indicated.

[57] For excellent treatment of medieval descriptions of leprosy as a venereal disease, see Whitwell, pp. 19–23, and especially Mettler, pp. 612 ff.

[58] *The questyonary of Cyrurgyens, with the formulary of lytell Guydo in Cyrurgie . . . newly Enprynted at London, by me Robert Wyer*, trans. Robert Copland (London, 1542), Q.ii. The passage is not found in the French text. See *La Grande Chirvrgie*, p. 405.

highly contagious disease which he too calls leprosy.[59] Richmond C. Holcomb concludes from an examination of early medical treatises that leprosy was always regarded as a readily contagious disease and that it was commonly believed to be contracted through venereal infection from a menstruous woman.[60]

Bartholomaeus Anglicus enumerates various causes of leprosy, and his text provides a convenient summary of the medieval understanding of the modes of infection.[61] It was of course true that leprosy was viewed not only as a venereal disease; the diversity of causes is almost staggering. Association with lepers, the bite of a venemous worm, unclean and corrupt wine, rotten meats and meats that easily rot, highly spiced meat—"as of long use of strong pepre and of garlyke," melancholic meat (too cold and dry), infected and corrupt air, the corrupt milk of a leprous wet nurse, the conception of a child "in menstrual tyme," and the infection of a child through father and mother "as it were by lawe of herytage" are among the causes listed by Barthelomeus. As he says, "Lepra cometh of dyvers causes . . . for the evil is contagious, and enfecteth other men." Near the head of his list, though, is the statement that "it cometh of flesshely lykynge by a womman soone after that a leprous man hath laye by her."

The medieval idea of sexual transmission is clearly not in keeping with the modern understanding of leprosy. Contemporary medicine states that infection may be the result of *prolonged* sexual contact; moreover, the long incubation period for leprosy makes it extremely difficult to locate the

[59] Whitwell, p. 52.
[60] *Who Gave the World Syphilis?* (New York, 1937), pp. 89–92.
[61] *De Proprietatibus Rerum*, book VII, chap. lxv.

source of infection confidently—to say that a woman who has slept with a leper can communicate the disease to a later and casual sexual partner. But medieval medicine makes exactly that statement. Whatever the treatise, one is likely to find in it that leprosy is spread through sexual intercourse or, more particularly, illicit sexual intercourse.

Since the tradition that viewed leprosy as a disease transmitted sexually was old and firmly established, it is not surprising that leprosy came to be associated with syphilis at the end of the fifteenth century. For instance, the traditional manner of representing leprosy in art was transferred to representations of syphilis. A late fifteenth-century pamphlet on the disease shows two patients, possibly a husband and wife, being examined by physicians, and both syphilitics are shown with skin markings reminiscent of those used in representations of lepers (fig. 11). A woodcut from the seventeenth century illustrates the treatment of syphilis with mercury, including by fumigation; a spotted syphilis patient is shown in the lower right-hand corner (fig. 12). Job—who during the Middle Ages was a patron of lepers[62]—becomes the patron saint of syphilis, which was also known as the *mal saint homme Job*.[63] During the late fifteenth and the sixteenth centuries, certain writers state that leprosy and syphilis are identical.[64] Paracelsus (1493–1541) writes that syphilis began with the combination of leprosy and another disease:

The French disease derives its origin from the coition of a leprous Frenchman with an impudent whore, who had venereal

[62] Riesman, *The Story of Medicine*, p. 311.

[63] Edmond Dupouy, *Le Moyen Age Médical* (Paris, 1895), p. 291.

[64] George Newman, "On the History of Leprosy," p. 64.

bubas, and after that infected everyone that lay with her; and thus from the leprosy and venereal bubas, the French disease arising, infected the whole world with its contagion, in the same manner as from coition of a horse and ass the race of mules is produced.[65]

Girolamo Fracastoro (1478–1553) comments on the confusion of syphilis and leprosy. He writes that many people equate elephantia and the French sickness because "the ancients wrote on leprosy and elephantia as two distinct diseases." Fracastoro points out that his mistaken contemporaries equate Greek leprosy (that is, scabies) with true leprosy and assume that elephantia must be syphilis, since they do not know what else it could be. Fracastoro asserts that elephantia should be equated with leprosy: "Elephantia is, strictly speaking, what is commonly called leprosy." He then proceeds to describe elephantia in detail and to distinguish it from syphilis. His presentation of elephantia is largely shaped by the same traditions that influence medieval accounts. For instance, he writes that

the nose becomes hollow, the mouth on both sides is stretched toward the ears, the eyes assume a rounded form and become like those of satyrs in paintings. Hence this disease has often been called "satyriasis" also; though some think that it is called satyriasis because of the abnormal sexual excitement that accompanies it. . . . Moreover the small blood vessels under the tongue become like varicose veins, the patient feels itching, and with it violent sexual excitement.[66]

[65] Quoted in Howard W. Haggard, *Devils, Drugs, and Doctors* (New York, 1929), pp. 245 f.

[66] Hieronymus Fracastorius, *De contagione et contagiosis morbis et eorum curatione, libri III*, ed. and trans. Wilmer Cave Wright (New York, 1930), pp. 158–163.

Thus, the sixteenth century, in the medieval tradition, acccepts leprosy as a readily contagious venereal disease linked with moral impurity. Not surprisingly, it associates leprosy with syphilis, and even when a writer such as Fracastoro seeks to differentiate the two diseases, he describes leprosy in terms used by medical writers of the Middle Ages. The symptom of sexual excitement—fancifully described hundreds of years earlier—is conventional at the end of the medieval period.

Medical treatises of the Middle Ages, which presented leprosy according to a fixed tradition, gave simple and strikingly similar accounts of signs and symptoms. Because the medical writer characteristically depended upon authorities rather than personal investigation, because his procedure was not empirical, he often described fanciful signs reported by his authorities. Even when he presented observable signs, he combined them into unrecognizable syndromes—particularly when the forms of leprosy discussed were linked with the humors. In short, the medieval physician was conditioned by authority and theory to describe leprosy inaccurately and unempirically. His accomplishment was profoundly important: he helped to shape the attitudes of his society, to create an atmosphere in which a disease, sufficiently horrible in itself, was viewed with unnecessary fear, loathing, and condemnation.

If no one had ever condemned the leper for his supposed moral impurity, he would nonetheless have been thought of with distaste because of his physical disfigurement. The fear of the disease is natural. However, medieval medicine helped turn that fear into an unnatural horror, for it could diagnose a multitude of diseases as leprosy. Let someone merely have gross skin lesions and he could be declared a leper. In a period when even the most aristocratic lived in filth and bathed irregularly, infection and disfiguring skin conditions were commonplace, and as a result so were diagnoses of leprosy.

Few misfortunes in medieval life were feared as much as such a diagnosis. It was a prediction of disfigurement and death, and what is perhaps more terrifying, it separated a man from society because of the infection he carried outwardly and the moral corruption that lay within him.

II

The Leper and Society

Now whosoever shall be defiled with the leprosy, and is separated by the judgment of the priest, shall have his clothes hanging loose, his head bare, his mouth covered with a cloth, and he shall cry out that he is defiled and unclean. All the time that he is a leper and unclean, he shall dwell alone without the camp.

Leviticus 13:44-46

Leprosy was more than just a disease to medieval man. It terrified him not only because its inevitable end was death, but even more because that death would be a long time in coming. The leper would suffer his disease for years, and so for years be at society's mercy. In one village, lepers might be bathed and fed but in another burned alive. There was a striking disparity between the stringency of laws enacted to contain the leper and the laxness with which they were enforced. If the leper's disease was feared for its contagiousness, and if edict upon edict was passed to prevent him from mingling with society, it is nonetheless true that he was often to be seen in the marketplace and on the road. The frequency with which laws were passed to restrict his mobility suggests that for all their harshness—and perhaps because of it—the laws were frequently unenforceable, or at least unenforced. Likewise the leper was by turns the object of vilification and of sympathy. A physician could assure the leper himself that his disease was a sign that God had chosen to grant his soul salvation, but he might simultaneously include in his diagnosis that his patient was morally corrupt. The Church might similarly decree that leprosy was a gift of God, but its bishops and priests would nonetheless use the disease as a metaphor for spiritual degeneration. The leper was seen as sinful and meritorious, as punished by God and as given special grace by Him.

Still, when one balances out this inconsistency and diversity of attitudes, the disease was for the most part considered a stigma, and the leper's existence was more often a living hell than the purgatory which his religion promised him.

The initiation of a victim into his hell was usually undertaken in an atmosphere of castigation. The law often required the leper to report himself to those entrusted with diagnosing leprosy, but voluntary admission of the disease must have been infrequent, and usually the separation of the leper began with public accusation by neighbors.[1] Then would follow a physical examination conducted by someone or some group considered expert on leprosy. In determining who ought to perform the diagnosis, the injunction in Leviticus was often observed. There it is stated that it is the duty of the priest to diagnose the disease and either pronounce the leper clean or separate him from society:

And the Lord spoke to Moses and Aaron, saying: The man in whose skin or flesh shall arise a different colour or a blister, or

[1] See the discussion later in this chapter of the expulsion of Jean Bodel; see also Jacques-Guy Cougoul, *La Lèpre dans l'Ancienne France* (Bordeaux, 1943), p. 32, and E. Jeanselme, "Comment l'Europe, au Moyen Age, se protégea contra la lèpre," *Bull Soc fr Hist Med*, XXV (1931), 34. Jeanselme's invaluable survey of the social position of the leper during the Middle Ages was of special value in the writing of this chapter.

as it were something shining, that is, the stroke of leprosy, shall be brought to Aaron the priest, or any one of his sons.[2]

The commandment is carried out in the New Testament. Matthew tells how Jesus cures a leper and then directs him to see a priest: "And Jesus saith to him, See thou tell no man; but go, shew thyself to the priest, and offer the gift which Moses commanded for a testimony unto them."[3] In Luke, Jesus directs ten lepers, "Go, shew yourselves to the priests" (17:14). In its turn, the medieval Church propagated the Levitical instructions.[4] For instance, in 1259 the Bishop of Amiens, Gerard de Conchy, echoed Leviticus 13:46 in stating that the segregation of lepers is divinely commanded: "Pius et misericors Dominus . . . leprosos manere precipit extra castra."[5] Thus, a suspected leper

[2] Leviticus 13:1–2 in the Douay-Rheims version, *The Holy Bible: Translated from the Latin Vulgate* (Baltimore, 1914). Cf. Deuteronomy 24:8: "Observe diligently that thou incur not the stroke of leprosy, but thou shalt do whatsoever the priests of the Levitical race shall teach thee, according to what I [Moses] have commanded them, and fulfil thou it carefully."

The following considerations have governed the choice of texts and translations of the Bible: translations of the New Testament and translations of the Old Testament which are intended to reflect the sense of the Vulgate text are taken from the Douay-Rheims version. Quotations of the Vulgate are taken from *Bibliorum Sacrorum iuxta Vulgatam Clementinam*, 2d ed., ed. Alosius Gramatica (Rome, 1959). Where the sense of the Hebrew must be conveyed, the following translations are used: published volumes of the Doubleday-Anchor Bible, and for books of the Pentateuch which have not yet appeared in Anchor Bible versions, the translation of the Torah published by the Jewish Publication Society.

[3] Matthew 8:4 in the Douay-Rheims version. Cf. Mark 1:44 and Luke 5:14.

[4] J. R. Whitwell, *Syphilis in Earlier Days* (London, 1940), p. 87.

[5] Cited by Paul Delaunay, "Histoire de la Médecine: De la con-

might be visited by a bishop or a competent person appointed by the bishop, such as a priest or ecclesiastical judge. In the matter of who should examine a suspect, there was no uniform procedure, however. In some parishes, an official tribunal summoned suspected lepers before it. For example, at Lille a tribunal of six lepers was given the responsibility of deciding whether an individual had leprosy and ought to be confined. The right to pronounce separation lay with the city magistrates at Amiens, with the bailiff at Piquigny, and with an abbot at Saint-Quentin.[6] To be sure, physicians also played a part in diagnosing lepers. Although in twelfth-century Cologne a group of three lepers diagnosed arrivals at the leprosarium, the responsibility for diagnosis was later assigned to the medical faculty.[7] As early as the fourteenth century, in Artois and Boulonnais, medical men were added to juries composed of lepers, and a century later practitioners took precedence over lepers. According to an ordinance dated 1500, the marquisate of Antwerp required a medical examination by six doctors and six or seven surgeons. However, the use of lepers and laymen as diagnosticians, or as consultants to physicians, was apparently widespread and retained at various places until the end of the leprosy period.[8] The process of examination in England apparently did not differ significantly from that on the continent: "Very much of the diagnosis of leprosy was left to the untrained and even

---

dition des lépreux au Moyen Age," *Hippocrate*, II (1934), 456. Cf. the Vulgate text: "Omni tempore, quo leprous est et immundus, solus habitabit extra castra." See also Numbers 5:1-2.

[6] Cougoul, pp. 61–62 and Jeanselme, pp. 34–35.

[7] Charles A. Mercier, *Leper Houses and Mediaeval Hospitals* (London, 1915), p. 11.

[8] Jeanselme, pp. 37–41.

uneducated. Diseases far removed from leprosy were doubt-less frequently classified with it. Gate porters, policemen, priests, and monks were frequently the judges in suspected cases."[9]

The physical examination of a suspected leper could come to one of four conclusions. The suspect could be de-clared healthy and given attestation that he was not leprous. Or, if the examiners thought that because of poor regimen the suspect might become leprous, he would be so ad-monished. If, however, the subject suffered a skin disease which could not be confirmed as leprosy, he would be confined to his home and strongly warned that he might have to enter a leper asylum if a later examination indi-cated the presence of leprosy. Finally, if the leprosy was confirmed, the victim would be told that he would have to be separated from the healthy population.[10]

In 1179, the Third Lateran Council issued a decree which urged that the segregation of lepers from society be accom-panied by appropriate ceremony. The decree provided a number of specimen rituals, and the *separatio leprosorum* in time came to be accepted widely, though not universally, for lepers continued to be treated with varying rigor. For instance, in England, where segregation was perhaps more lax than elsewhere, the ceremony of the symbolic burial

[9] George Newman, "On the History of the Decline and Final Extinction of Leprosy as an Endemic Disease in the British Is-lands," *Prize Essays on Leprosy*, The New Sydenham Society, CLVII (London, 1895), 56. See also, Whitwell, p. 87; Rotha Mary Clay, *The Medieval Hospitals of England* (London, 1909), p. 59; Richmond C. Holcomb, *Who Gave the World Syphilis?* (New York, 1937), p. 71; Cougoul, pp. 61–62.

[10] Jeanselme, p. 50.

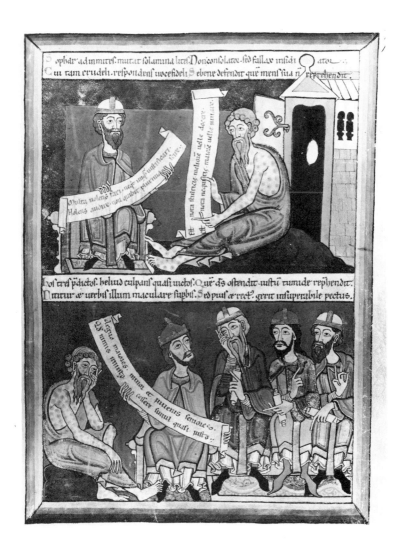

1. Job with Zophar (top panel); with his comforters (bottom panel). Gregory, *Moralia in Job* (late twelfth century). Paris. Bibliothèque Nationale. MS. Latin 15675, fol. 7 recto.

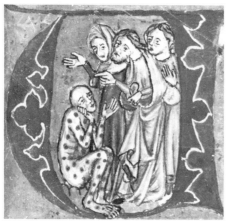

2. Job and his comforters. Paraphrase of the Book of Job (German, fourteenth century). Gottingen. Staatliches Archivlager, Staatsarchiv Königsberg (Archivbestände Preussischer Kulturbesitz). MS. A 191, fol. 421.

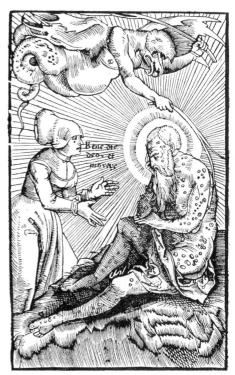

3. Job's wife urging him to bless God and die. Woodcut by Hans Wechbelin for Hans von Gerssdorff's *Feldbuch der Wundarznei* (Strasbourg, 1517). The Bettman Archive.

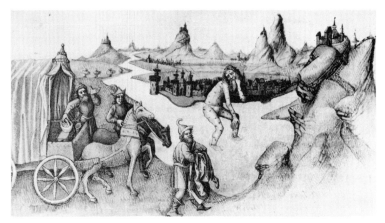

4. Naaman the leper bathing in the Jordan (German, fifteenth century). The Bettmann Archive.

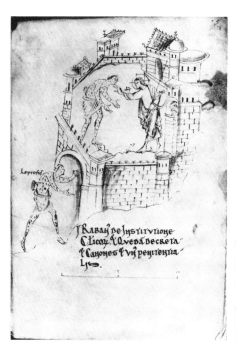

Leprosus

¶Rabah de institutione
Clicorū Queda decreta
T canones ī vñ penitentia
Ls.

5. Jesus healing a leper. Gospel book from the abbey at Essen; originally from Coblenz, possibly from the monastery of St. Florinus (second half of ninth century). Dusseldorf. Landesbildstelle Rheinland. MS. Cod. B. 113, fol. 5 recto.

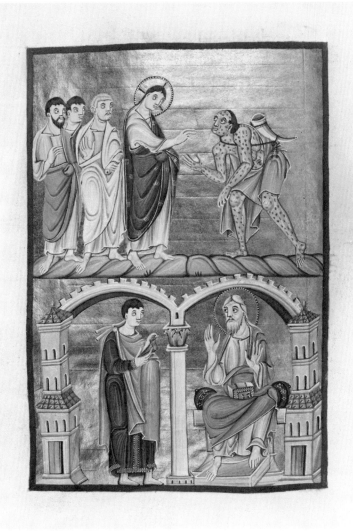

6. Jesus, with Peter and two other apostles, healing a leper (top panel); the cured leper bearing two doves to a priest (bottom panel). Gospel Book of Otto III (ca. 1000). Munich. Bayerische Staatsbibliothek. MS. Latin 4453, fol. 97 verso.

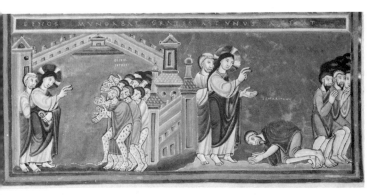

7. Jesus healing the ten lepers, only one of whom returns to glorify him (Luke 17:12–19). Echternach Gospel Book (1020–1030). Nurenberg. Germanisches Nationalmuseum. MS. 156142, fol. 55 verso (bottom panel).

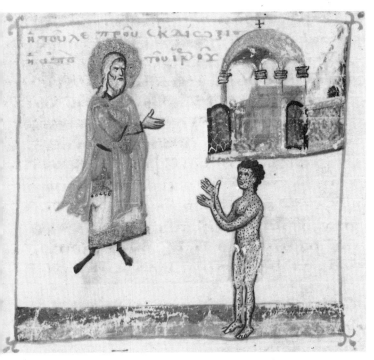

8. Aaron and a leper. *Octateuch* (thirteenth century). Rome. Biblioteca Apostolica Vaticana. MS. gr. 746, fol. 281 recto.

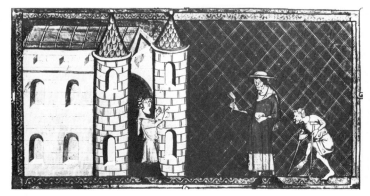

9. Josaphat as a child, meeting a leper and a cripple at the gates of Jerusalem. Vincent of Beauvais, *Miroir Historial* (fourteenth century). Paris. Bibliothèque de l'Arsenal. MS. 5080. The Bettmann Archive.

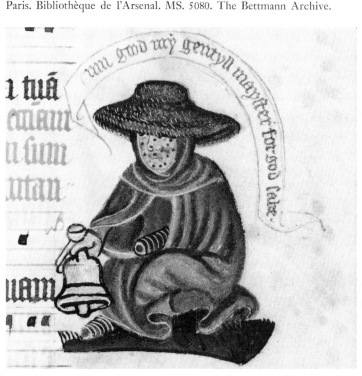

10. A leper seeking alms. Exeter Pontifical (late fourteenth or early fifteenth century). London. British Museum. MS. Lans. 451, fol. 127.

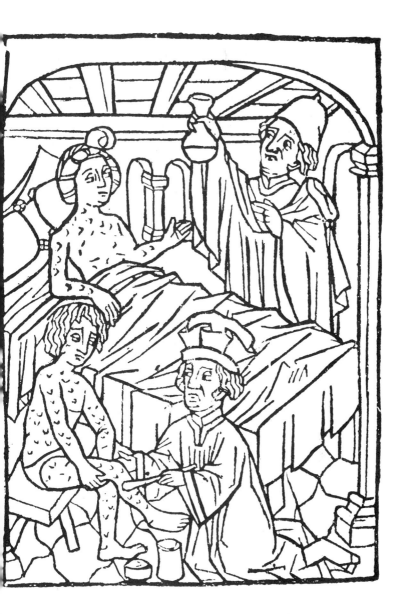

11. Doctors examining and treating syphilitics. Woodcut from the title page of Bartholomeus Steber's *A malafranczos morbo gallorum* . . . (Vienna, 1497–1498). The Bettmann Archive.

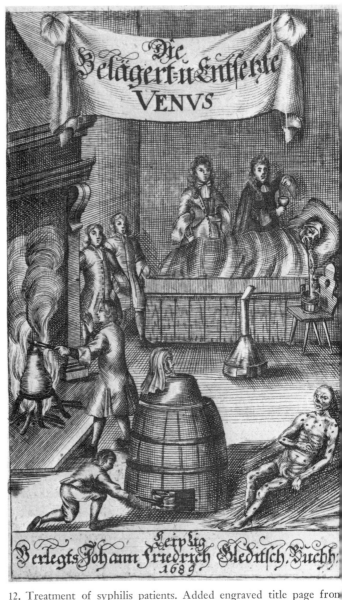

12. Treatment of syphilis patients. Added engraved title page from
Steven Blankaart, *Die belägert-und entsetzte Venus* (Leipzig, 1689)
National Library of Medicine, Bethesda, Maryland 20014.

service was not in force.[11] Moreover, even where the ritual
was followed, there was no uniformity of procedure; the
ceremonies differed with time and place, so that several of
them stipulate changes in procedures established in earlier
rituals.[12] Nonetheless, in France, Flanders, and the south
side of the Rhine—that is, in all the territory of ancient
Gaul—the rituals of separation were similar. In removing
the leper from the world, the ceremonies differed little
from the office for the dead, for in principle the leper was
no longer one of the living.[13] The Church recognized that
the steps it required were severe, even cruel, but out of
fear of contagion, it set out to enforce isolation. For instance, a council held at Lavaur, in the south of France,
issued the following edict:

One may have very great compassion for the victims, and one
may embrace them with fraternal charity—those unfortunates
who, by the will of God, are tormented by leprosy; but because this illness is contagious, wishing to prevent danger, we
command that lepers be sequestered from the rest of the faithful; that they do not enter any public place—churches, mar-
kets, public squares, inns; that their clothing be uniform, their
beards and hair shaved; they shall have a special burial place,
and shall always carry a signal by which one can recognize
them.[14]

[11] William MacArthur "Medieval 'Leprosy' in the British Isles,"
Leprosy Rev, XXIV (1953), 12.
[12] Jeanselme, pp. 3, 35; and Rud. Virchow, "Zur Geschichte des
Aussatzes und der Spitäler, besonders in Deutschland: Vierter
Artikel," *Arch path Anat Physiol*, XX (1861), 167.
[13] Cougoul, pp. 66 f. and Jeanselme, pp. 62 f.
[14] *Concilium Vaurense* (1368), canon 21, in *Sacrorum conciliorum nova et amplissima collectio*, ed. Phil. Labbeus et al., XXVI
(Graz, 1961), 499.

The sequestration of lepers was carried out with appropriate solemnity. Jeanselme outlines a representative office of separation by synthesizing rituals followed in seventeen dioceses (pp. 63 ff.). During the ceremony, the leper knelt before the altar, beneath a black cloth supported by two trestles. (However, at Amiens and elsewhere, he was required to stand in a grave in a cemetery.) His face was covered by a black veil as he heard the mass. The officiating priest threw a spadeful of earth from the cemetery on the head of the leper three times, explaining that the ritual symbolizes the death of the leper to the world. The priest said: "Be dead to the world, be reborn to God," and the leper replied, "O Jesus, my redeemer, you formed me out of earth, you dressed me in a body; let me be reborn in the final day."[15] Then, using the vernacular, the priest read the prohibitions that made the alienation of the victim explicit:

I forbid you to ever enter the church or monastery, fair, mill, marketplace, or company of persons. I forbid you to ever leave your house without your leper's costume, in order that one recognize you and that you never go barefoot. I forbid you to wash your hands or any thing about you in the stream or in the fountain and to ever drink; and if you wish water to drink, fetch it in your cask or porringer. I forbid you to touch anything you bargain for or buy, until it is yours. I forbid you to enter a tavern. If you want wine, whether you buy it or someone gives it to you, have it put in your cask. I forbid you to live with any woman other than your own. I forbid you, if you go on the road and you meet some person who speaks

[15] *Ex antiquo Rituali insignis ecclesiae Catalaunensis* (n.d.), in *De antiquis Ecclesiae ritibus libri ex variis insigniorum Ecclesiarum . . .* , ed. Edmond Martène, vol. III (Antwerp, 1737), cols. 1013-1014.

to you, to fail to put yourself downwind before you answer. I forbid you to go in a narrow lane, so that should you meet any person, he should not be able to catch the affliction from you. I forbid you, if you go along any thoroughfare, to ever touch a well or the cord unless you have put on your gloves. I forbid you to ever touch children or to give them anything. I forbid you to eat or drink from any dishes other than your own. I forbid you drinking or eating in company, unless with lepers.[16]

Following the reading of the proscriptions, the leper put on his costume and was given the signal with which he was to warn the healthy of his approach.[17] Both signal and costume varied with locality. The instrument for warning the populace of the leper's approach was usually a rattle or castanet, but it was sometimes a bell, either carried or worn on the shoes. At Lille, the leper carried a small horn, and at Arles he sang the "De Profundis" to warn the healthy of his presence. As for his clothing, he usually wore gloves and long robes. In certain areas, the costumes were distinguished by cut or color (for example, white was worn in Poitiers, grey or black with an embroidered red letter *L* in France), though in England there was little uniformity.[18] In figure 9, a leper is shown in traditional costume and carrying traditional gear: he wears gloves and a long robe, and he carries a clapper in one hand and a bowl in the other. The seated leper in figure 10 is also in a long robe but carries a bell. The lepers in figures 5 and 6 wear horns over their shoulders.

[16] *Ex veteri codice S. Albini Andegavensis* (n.d.), in Martène, cols. 1005–1006.

[17] Jeanselme, p. 63.

[18] Patrick Feeny, *The Fight against Leprosy* (London, 1964), p. 30.

Equipped with his clothing and various utensils, the leper would be led to his place of retreat, often a hut situated in an open field outside of the town. At the threshhold of his hut, the leper had to say, "This retreat is mine, I will live here always because I have chosen it."[19] The priest would bless the outcast's utensils and encourage him to be patient. The ritual of St. Albin d'Angers directs the cleric to say:

Because of greatly having to suffer sadness, tribulation, disease, leprosy, and other worldly adversity, one reaches the kingdom of paradise, where there is neither disease nor adversity, but all are pure and spotless, without filth and without any stain of filth, more resplendent than the sun, where you will go, if it please God. But so that you be a good Christian and so that you bear this adversity patiently, God gives you grace.[20]

In the ritual of separation used at Reims, the priest consoles the leper that even if he is separated from the healthy,

this separation is only corporeal; as for the spirit, which is uppermost, you will always be as much as you ever were and will have part and portion of all the prayers of our mother Holy Church, as if every day you were a spectator at the divine service with others. And concerning your small necessities, people of means will provide them, and God will never forsake you. Only take care and have patience. God be with you.[21]

The priest would next place a cross before the leper's door, hang a box for alms on the cross, and place an offering in it, at the same time admonishing those gathered for the ceremony not to injure the leper by word or action, but rather—having a remembrance of the human condition and

[19] Jeanselme, p. 67.
[20] *Ex veteri codice S. Albini Andegavensis*, in Martène, col. 1005.
[21] *Ex Rituali ad usum provinciae Remensis* (n.d.), in Martène, col. 1009.

the formidable judgment of God—to provide liberally for all his needs. The congregation would presumably follow the priest's example and place alms in the leper's cup. Finally, the priest advised parents, or whoever was in guardianship of the leper, to remain close to him for at least thirty-two hours in order to provide comfort and assistance if the leper were to enter a physical or spiritual crisis. The leper was now separated from the world.

In general outline, at least, this was the procedure used in sequestering lepers in a large portion of Europe. Deviations from the procedure of course occurred. On the one hand, the lepers were sometimes dealt with brutally and murdered outright:

Several highly placed lepraphobes, including Henry II of England, his great-grandson Edward I, and Philip V of France, took the position that the recommended ritual was unnecessarily symbolical. The revisions instituted by Henry and Philip were similar. Both chose to replace the religious service with a simple civil ceremony. It consisted of strapping the leper to a post and setting him afire. Edward adhered a trifle more closely to the letter of the ecumenical decree. Lepers, during his reign, were permitted the comforts of a Christian funeral. They were led down to the cemetery and buried alive.[22]

On the other hand, for some of the afflicted, it was possible to be neither murdered nor sent to a leper asylum. Those with money could chose to enter certain institutions which, although not leprosariums, accepted lepers. Thus, although in theory all lepers, whatever their social status, were liable

[22] Berton Roueché, "A Lonely Road," in *Eleven Blue Men: And Other Narratives of Medical Detection* (New York, 1953), p. 117.

to be isolated in asylums, in practice there were many exceptions, and these were usually persons of rank or wealth. A privileged leper could obtain permission to remain outside the leprosarium, either secluded in his own home or in a house or small farm in the countryside.[23] And even were he made to enter a leper house, the situation could be made bearable for a person of position. The leper asylum frequently granted such individuals the right to construct (at their own expense) a building on the leprosarium's land,[24] and certain leprosariums were even reserved exclusively for stipulated classes: "In Dauphigne there was one leper house for the commons, another for the nobles, and a third for ladies of the Court. The hospital at Walsingham was for lepers who were rich and of good family and that of St. Lawrence at Canterbury for the clergy."[25]

Nonetheless, even at their best, the asylums were by their very nature constant reminders of the hopelessness of the

---

[23] An instance of this is seen in Hartmann von Aue's *Der Arme Heinrich*. Heinrich voluntarily isolates himself on a woodland farm (see Chapter IV). This is but one example of how medieval poetry reflects contemporary conditions. Detailed studies of the historical basis for descriptions of lepers in literature are to be found in Pierre Jonin, *Les Personnages féminins dans les romans français de Tristan au XIIe siècle: Étude des influences contemporains*, Publication des annales de la faculté des lettres, Aix-en-Provence, new series, no. 22 (Gap, 1958), pp. 109–138; Paul Remy, "La lèpre, thème littéraire au moyen âge: Commentaire d'un passage du roman provençal de Jaufré," *MA*, LII (1946), 195–242; Wilhelm Wackernagel, "Abhandlung," in *Der Arme Heinrich Herrn Hartmanns von Aue und Zwei Jüngere Prosalegenden Verwandten Inhaltes*, ed. Wilhelm Wackernagel and Ernst Stadler (Basel, 1911), pp. 189–243. Of the three studies, Wackernagel's is the most comprehensive.

[24] Jeanselme, pp. 70–72.

[25] Mercier, pp. 18 f. See also Cougoul, pp. 95 ff.

leper's plight. It is true that the diagnostician's decision could be appealed and that internment was not necessarily lifelong. For instance, incarceration might be relaxed during lulls in epidemics—that is, when the disease ceased being endemic. Moreover, if the unlikely did happen, if a victim's symptoms vanished, he could be released. There is a record of one such case from the middle of the fifteenth century. A patient who was seen to be healthy was discharged, but he later showed new symptoms and was recommitted. After four weeks of treatment, he was returned to his family.[26] But healing of the disease must have been extremely rare. Guy of Chauliac writes:

It is agreed by all that leprosy is a very injurious disease, and that it is hereditary and contagious, and is almost impossible to eradicate, especially confirmed [leprosy]. For how (says Avicenna) should leprosy be cured, being an extensive canker (*chancre universel*), seeing that a confined canker (*chancre particulier*) can not be healed. It may well be endured and alleviated, but not healed. Moreover, it is agreed that among the varieties of leprosy, leonine and elephantic (as very injurious matter) are the worst: the others, as more treatable, are more gentle.[27]

Medicine, such as it was, held out little hope to the diseased man. Essentially, no therapy was available to the leper, and prophylaxis consisted merely of isolation.[28] Remedies were boasted, but most of these were unattainable and ineffectual. The proposed cures were, like most reme-

[26] Jeanselme, pp. 61 f. Mercier, pp. 10 f., alludes to two similar events.

[27] Guy of Chauliac, *La Grande Chirvrgie*, ed. E. Nicaise (Paris, 1890), p. 406.

[28] Cougoul, p. 30.

dies until the nineteenth century, often bizarre and fantastic. Alchemy, and particularly the gold of the alchemist, could purify the leper; so could the earth from an anthill, or the perfumed water in which the Christ child had been washed, or His swaddling clothes, or the blood of a turtle from the Cape Verde Islands,[29] or the blood of an infant.[30] One collection of medical recipes contains the following prescription:

Also a principal medicine for leprosy. Take a bushel of good barley in the month of March, and half a bushel of toads; and seethe them well together in a lead [cauldron] with running water, till bones of the toads be altogether shaken out; then take out the barley from the water, and dry [it] in the sun or in a kiln till it be right dry. Then take a hen that hath chickens new-hatched, that have never eaten food; and put them in a close house [coop] clean swept, and give them of the barley broken in a mortar and afterwards whole when they are older; then let the leper eat those chickens both roasted and boiled, and no other meat; and let his bread be made of barley and [his] drink scalded, and ever-among [from time to time] drink water, ale, and wine, but scalded, nor any hot nor spiced drink, and ever-among let the blood till thou seest thy blood

[29] Lynn Thorndike, *A History of Magic and Experimenal Science*, 8 vols. (New York, 1923–1958), III, 630; II, 147; I, 390, 392; IV, 546.

[30] There is evidence that physicians did sometimes recommend the blood of human children as a cure for leprosy. See Remy, pp. 221–223. Nevertheless, there is no evidence that the procedure was ever widely suggested or adopted; rather, the practice of sacrificing children for their blood seems to have been confined primarily to literary texts, where the use of blood of innocent children to cure a moral disease had symbolical value. See Chapter IV, n. 5.

clean. And govern thee in all things as it be aforesaid, and thou shalt be whole. *Probatum est.*[31]

The Bible has its cures as well. The soldier Naaman—"he was a valiant man and rich, but a leper"—dips himself in the Jordan seven times according to the advice of Elisha and is immediately cleansed.[32] Luke tells how Jesus directs ten lepers to "shew yourselves to the priests." The lepers leave, but they are purified before they come to the priests.[33] In Matthew, "a leper came and adored [Jesus], saying, Lord, if thou wilt, thou canst make me clean. And Jesus stretching forth his hand touched him, saying: I will, be thou made clean. And forthwith his leprosy was cleansed."[34] However, since the medieval leper could not count on a miraculous cure, the diagnosis of his disease was usually a prediction of lifelong suffering and isolation.

The asylums which confined the leper were intended to assure his separation. Nearly always, they were located outside cities and towns, away from centers of human

---

[31] *A Leechbook or Collection of Medical Recipes of the Fifteenth Century*, ed. and trans. Warren R. Dawson (London, 1934), pp. 183, 185.

[32] II Kings 5. Unlike other cures in the Bible, Naaman's is not necessarily miraculous. Until relatively recently leprosy was regularly confused with other conditions; Naaman's healing suggests he was actually afflicted with scabies, "which is still cured by bathing in the sulphurous springs of the Jordan valley." See Ernest Muir, *Manual of Leprosy* (Baltimore, 1948), p. 3. For an analogue to Naaman's cure, see Lee S. Huizinga, "Leprosy in Legend and History: King Bladud of England," *Leper Quart*, XIII (1939), 18–20. Bladud heals himself in the hot springs of a swamp, and then founds the city of Bath at the spot. In 1138, the Bishop of Bath built a leprosarium there at one of the springs.

[33] Luke 17:11–19.

[34] Matthew 8:2–3. Cf. Mark 1:40–42 and Luke 5:12–13.

activity, and should the town expand around it, the leprosarium would be moved. At Rostock, Cologne, and other places, the leprosariums were situated at the site where executions of criminals were held. Whenever possible, the asylums were built downwind from the town, so that the prevailing wind did not pass first over the leprosarium and then over the town.[35]

In its simplest form, the asylum a village would build for one leper would be a small wooden cottage, elevated on four props and surrounded by a fence. When the diseased were numerous, their huts and the cultivated land around the buildings would be located in an enclosure. The Third Lateran Council provided that asylums of this size should have their own chapel, cemetery, and priest. In time, stone buildings might be constructed, either on the same plan as the wooden huts or else much larger and divided into small cubicles for individual lepers. Within a single leprosarium, the rich could live in private dwellings while the poor were crowded together.[36]

By the thirteenth century, the asylum at Reims was this kind of elaborate leprosarium. Most of the asylum's land was given over to farming, and so a cowshed, a sheepfold, a barn, an enclosure for pigs, and other farm buildings were on the property. The community, which had two groups of brethren (the lepers and the members of religious orders), lived in two separate buildings. The lepers' building had a kitchen and a refectory; the refectory, which also served as sleeping quarters, had a fireplace and eight beds. The lepers had a courtyard in which it was possible to walk when it rained, and a garden. In addition, they had their

[35] Jeanselme, pp. 73–75.
[36] Jeanselme, pp. 75–81.

own cemetery and chapel. Two structures originally built
by lepers early in the fourteenth century became the property of the asylum at their owners' deaths. A similar complex existed about one mile away for female lepers.[37]

It is difficult to give a blanket description of life inside
an asylum, to say whether the lepers were cared for or
were brutalized, but certain generalizations can be offered.
In their intent, at least, the asylums were established to confine lepers (and so the disease) and to keep them alive:

Leper houses were hospitals in the sense that they were institutions for the reception of the sick, and in some leper houses
there were nurses to dress the sores of the lepers; but on the
whole, leper houses were rather combinations of the prison,
the monastery, and the almshouse than hospitals in the modern
sense. The primary function of the leper house was to form a
prison, or, if we prefer the term, a compulsory isolation hospital, for the seclusion of the lepers from the general population.[38]

At the outset, the Church seems to have undertaken the
responsibility of establishing and maintaining leprosariums;
in the sixth century, the Councils of Orleans and Lyons
"decided that lepers ought to be kept at the expense of the
Church, and under the care of the bishops."[39] In time, how-

[37] Paul Hildenfinger, *La Léproserie de Reims du XIIe au XVIIe
siècle* (Reims, 1906), pp. 20–23.

[38] Mercier, p. 7. Loren C. MacKinney, *Early Medieval Medicine:
With Special Reference to France and Chartres* (Baltimore, 1937),
pp. 176 f., states that early (sixth to eighth century) medieval
leprosariums belong to that class of medieval institutions established "for general charity and with provision for the care (*cura*)
of the sick inmates, but not for the active cure of diseases." In the
centuries following, little occurred to alter the operations of the
asylums.

[39] Mercier, p. 8.

ever, control of the asylums became increasingly secular, particularly in Germany, where in early times the conduct of the hospitals took on a more nonreligious character than in France, where Church organization was retained until quite late.[40] Usually, the bishops appointed administrators for the leper houses, but occasionally (as in fourteenth century Paris) they would manage them personally, taking financial, disciplinary, and other control.[41] Nonetheless, in France also the control of the asylums gradually became secular. At Reims, for example, the leprosarium was initially (that is, before the middle of the twelfth century) under the control of the archbishop, but within one hundred years the administration had passed to the city magistrates. In 1231, two members of the laity were entrusted with being headmasters, a practice which the archbishop confirmed in 1240, after which the direct administration became the responsibility of the municipal government.[42]

In Church-controlled leper houses, the hospitalers lived according to codes based upon the rule of Saint Augustine, which they adapted to their particular needs. In 1212 and 1214 the Councils of Paris and Rouen attempted to establish one rule for all hospitals and leprosariums having a religious congregation. Several fundamental principles were set down, among them the requirements that all residents of leprosariums take the vows of poverty, chastity, and obedience; that they all wear the religious habit; and that those wishing to be maintained at the expense of the house without accepting the obligations of religious life be

[40] Virchow, p. 168.
[41] Cougoul, pp. 89–92.
[42] Hildenfinger, pp. 5–6.

excluded. After a few years, the prescriptions of the councils came to be applied at particular establishments.[43]

Seclusion in a leprosarium—particularly one governed by religious rule—must have exacted an enormous emotional payment from the inmates. In a religious leprosarium, to the inevitable sense of mortality were added the burdens and discipline of an ascetic life. For instance, the lepers of the asylum at Illeford took the monastic vows of poverty, chastity, and obedience; and in 1346, the Bishop of London directed that they

omit not attendance at divine service unless prevented by grievous bodily infirmity; they are to preserve silence there, and to hear matins and mass throughout if they are able, and while there to be intent on prayer and devotion. Every leper shall say every day for morning duty a paternoster and an ave thirteen times, and for the other hours of the day respectively, viz., the first, third, and sixth hours, the hour of vespers, and again at compline, a paternoster and an ave seven times; and besides the aforesaid prayers, each leprous brother shall say a pater and an ave thirty times every day for the founders, and for the bishop, and for all the benefactors of the hospital, and for all true believers, living and dead; and on the day on which any of the brothers depart this life, let each brother say in addition fifty paters and aves three times for the souls of the departed and of all deceased true believers. And if anyone shall openly transgress the said rules, for each transgression let him suffer punishment according to the gravity of his offense from the Master, but if secretly, let him be dealt with by the priest in the penitential court.[44]

[43] Léon Le Grand, ed., *Statuts d'hotels-dieu et de léproseries: Recueil de textes du XIIe au XIVe siècle* (Paris, 1901), pp. v–viii, xii–xiii.

[44] Quoted in Mercier, pp. 27–28. See also p. 16.

If the rules that governed leper houses at all accurately depict what life in the houses was like, existence in an asylum must have been generally grim and disciplined. The statutes dictated what kind of clothing and furniture the leper might have. They fixed limits within which the leper could roam, even within the asylum. He could be forbidden to approach the kitchen, the church choir, the women's quarters, the barn, the food storeroom, the garden, the well. The statutes set up punishments for offenses, such as assault and battery, fornication, sleeping outside the leprosarium, touching ecclesiastical ornaments. They controlled his amusements by forbidding drinking, chess, dice playing, and other gambling. They required the leper to turn his goods over to the leprosarium and threatened him with excommunication for failing to do so. They forbad him to marry, or allowed him to marry only another leper, or required him to leave the leprosarium if he did marry, or if he was married they forbad him to live with his wife.[45] In short, mortification of the spirit and mortification of the flesh were the consequence of the rule. And if in practice the rules were not followed closely, still they were always there as the expression of an attitude of the society which excluded the leper. For example, at the leprosarium at St. Albans, the first injunction of "a book of rules drawn up for the guidance of its inmates" stipulates:

Amongst all infirmities, the disease of leprosy may be considered the most loathsome, and those who are smitten with it ought at all times, and in all places, as well in their conduct as in their dress, to bear themselves as more to be despised and as more humble than all other men.[46]

[45] Le Grand, p. 181 et passim.
[46] Quoted in Roueché, p. 115. For the Latin (written 1335–1349), see *Articuli observandi inter Fratres professos Domus Sancti*

The demand that the leper abase himself is the expression of a moral judgement, of a need to exclude the leper, of fear. The leper was a threat to society, the carrier of contagion, and society did what it could to protect itself. It was perhaps an unintentional byproduct that in protecting society by isolating the leper, the leper was sometimes protected from society by being isolated. What could an ordinary man who became a leper do once his disease could no longer be hidden? He could not easily practice a trade, for few would deal with him. Perhaps the best he could expect would be to remain isolated in his own home and dependent upon family or friends for maintenance. What often happened was that he became a beggar totally reliant upon the rare good will of other men. An early description of lepers—given in a funeral sermon in 379 by St. Gregory of Nazianzus—portrays what the unconfined leper could expect at any era. Gregory describes lepers as

men already dead except to sin; often dumb, with festering bodies whose insensible limbs rotted off them; heartbreaking and horrifying spectacles of human ruin; objects of repugnance and terror; driven from the house, the marketplace, the village, and the fountain; persecuted even by their parents; disfigured, unrecognisable, identified only by their names; avoided, shrunk from, detested, despised by relatives, fathers, mothers, spouses, children; wandering night and day, naked, destitute, exposing their loathsomeness to the gaze of passers-by to move them and obtain alms.[47]

Juliani, juxta Sanctum Albanum, "Appendix C," *Gesta Abbatum Sancti Albani,* ed. Henry Thomas Riley, II (London, 1867), 503.

[47] Quoted in Mercier, p. 5. For the Latin, see "Oratio XLIII: In laudem Basilii Magni," LXIII (*PG,* XXXVI, 579). The reference here is to a work in the *Patrologia Graeca,* ed. J. P. Migne, 162 vols. (Paris, 1857–1866); cf. Chapter III, n. 28.

And St. Gregory of Nysse (332–400), in the middle of a detailed description of the physical ravages of leprosy, defines the lepers' relationship to society:

They have no friends but each other, united as they are in misery; that which makes them despised of others unites them in a close bond among themselves; repulsed on all sides, they become by their union a people in themselves . . . Are they not excluded from public assemblies and feastdays like murderers, parricides, fated to be perpetual exiles, and even more unhappy than these! For murderers are at least permitted to live with other men; these are driven away like enemies. They are denied the same roof, the same table, the same utensils with others. Moreover they are barred from the cleansing waters for public usage, and there is fear that even the rivers may be infected with their malady. If a dog should lap water with a wounded tongue, we should not consider the water to have been contaminated by the brute; but let one of these afflicted ones approach it and we believe the water is rendered impure by this human being.[48]

The leper's situation was almost unendurable, for he was not only at the mercy of other men, but also at the mercy of the law. Physical conditions—for example, infancy, lunacy, and leprosy—endowed persons with special forms of status,[49] but no other condition had a legal status as appalling as that of leprosy. For instance, in 643, Rothar —the Lombard King—issued the following decree:

If anyone becomes a leper, and this becomes known to a judge

[48] M. Webster Brown, "Two Ancient Descriptions of Lepers," *Med J Rec*, CXXXVII (1933), 299. For the original passage, see *De pauperibus amandis, oratio II*, in PG, XLVI, 477–478.
[49] W. S. Holdsworth, *A History of English Law*, 3d ed., III (Boston, 1927), 457.

or a matter of general repute to the people, and he is expelled from his city or dwelling, so that he lives alone, let him not be permitted to give or donate his possessions to anyone at all, because on the very day when he is expelled, he is considered as dead. Nevertheless, as long as he lives let him be supported from the possesions he leaves, for good will.[50]

The principle voiced in Rothar's edict was elaborated and persisted for many years after him. In a study of French civil law, one legal historian takes note of the juridical tradition that declared the leper dead. In thirteenth-century Beauvoisis the law was explicit: the leper is dead to the world, "il est mort quant au siècle." From the day of his separation, he lost all right of ownership and his estate from that time onward was unprotected. On the other hand, in Normandy, the leper was allowed to retain his possessions, or at least to have the usufruct of them. Nevertheless, he could neither make a will nor inherit goods. At Ypres, a leper admitted to the asylum was required to turn all of his property over to it if he had no wife or children, or in the event that he had family, a certain part of his wealth was given to the sanatorium. Any wealth inherited by him after his separation from society belonged to the asylum. In contrast, at Hainaut, the leper was permitted to inherit and to bequeath property, and at Noyon a will could be made with the authorization of the master of the leprosarium. However, it was more typical that the leper was denied all or part of the privileges of ownership.[51]

[50] *Edictum Rotharis regis CLXXVI*, cited in Latin by Jeanselme, p. 138, and with some minor differences in Vincenzo d'Amato, *La Lebbre nella Storia, nella Geografia e nell'Arte* (Rome, 1923), p. 29, n. 1.

[51] Paul Viollet, *Droit privé et sources: Histoire du droit civil français*, 2d ed. (Paris, 1893), pp. 375–376.

French legal custom had analogues in England, where the law was similarly inconsistent. As in France, the leper could be permitted to leave property,[52] but by and large the privilege was not granted to him. In 1200, the Provincial Synod of Westminster denied lepers the right to make a will, to inherit property, or to plead in a common law court.[53] For their part, the courts tended to uphold the principle that leprosy denies a leper the usual rights of ownership. In one instance, bequests made by a leper were deemed invalid because they were made before the king's direction concerning disposal of the property; the leper's property was turned over to someone outside his family.[54] In 1223, a case was brought to court in Suffolk by Salomon of Wepstede, who claimed to have been given a parcel of land by John before John had been turned out of the community because of his leprosy. However, John's daughter Maria and her husband Thomas denied Salomon's right to the property, claiming that John was a leper when the grant was made. The court directed that if Maria and Thomas could prove their contention, Salomon would have no right to the property.[55] In 1227, in the county court of Hereford, a woman named Agnes, the wife of John of Westwick, sought to initiate legal action to obtain property

[52] William MacAruthur, "Some Notes on Old-Time Leprosy in England and Ireland," *J Roy Army Med Corps*, XLV (1925), 413.

[53] Newman, p. 33.

[54] Newman, p. 14.

[55] Henry de Bracton, *Bracton's Note Book: A Collection of Cases Decided in the King's Courts during the Reign of Henry the Third*, ed. F. W. Maitland (London, 1887), III, 502–503. "[In Bracton's treatise] the law set forth is the custom of England as developed by central royal courts" (Munroe Smith, *The Development of European Law* [New York, 1928], p. 248).

willed her by her husband. However, because she was a leper, the court prevented her from suing for the dower, although it allowed her to keep the property she owned before John died.[56] Thus, in medieval English law, "the leper is excommunicate in a very real sense. He is put outside the community of mankind; the place for him is the lazar house. Not only is he incapable of suing and of making gifts or contracts, but he is even incapable of inheriting. He still remains the owner of what he was before his 'segregation,' but he can not inherit."[57]

The leper's legal status made him susceptible to terrible injustices. As Cougoul points out (p. 32), since the leper often had no right to make a will, his property sometimes went to the *seigneur*. Thus, in any locality where the leper lost the privileges both of retaining and distributing his estate, a person might be put in a leper house so that the *seigneur* could gain profit or vengeance. In another form of injustice, an asylum might have its experts decide that a suspected case was not leprosy if its facilities would be strained by yet one more sufferer, particularly if the victim could not afford to buy his way into the community of afflicted.[58]

The anguish of a person about to be examined for leprosy must have been beyond measure, for a positive finding could not only deprive him of his property but also of his spouse—though here again the situation varied from place to

[56] Henry de Bracton, *Henrici de Bracton De legibus & consuetudinibus Angliae* (London, 1569), fol. 421, tract. 3.

[57] Frederick Pollock and Frederic William Maitland, *The History of English Law before the Time of Edward I*, 2d ed., I (Cambridge, Eng., 1899), 480.

[58] Delaunay, p. 457, and Jeanselme, p. 37.

place and time to time. At the close of the fourth century Pope Sirice permitted divorce if a healthy man married a leper (or a woman who subsequently became leprous) and the union produced none but leprous children.[59] One of Rothar's laws (643) provides a typical formulation of the sort of law which named leprosy as an obstacle to marriage. The law states that if an engaged woman becomes leprous (or demoniac or blind as a result of sin), the fiancé is permitted to take back his marriage portion and break the engagement without fear of a lawsuit:

If it happens that after becoming engaged, a girl or woman becomes leprous, demoniac, or blind in both eyes through sin, then the fiancé may take back his goods and ought not be forced to accept her for a wife on compulsion, nor should any charge be laid against him for such cause, because it was not his fault but was due to the presence of sin and the access of sickness.[60]

In 757, the Parliament of Compiègne, under Pépin le Bref, authorized a leper to permit a healthy spouse to remarry, though at about the same time Pope Stephen II "refused to sanction divorce on this ground."[61]

In general, the Church did not hold that leprosy stood in the way of marriage. The Third Lateran Council decreed that if a leper did not wish to live in continence and if he found a woman who would marry him, they could

[59] Jeanselme, p. 12.

[60] *Leges Rotharis, CLXXX,* cited by Jeanselme, p. 138, and d'Amato, p. 29, n. 1.

[61] Mercier, p. 15. The edict of the Parliament is quoted in Auguste Harmand, *Notice historique sur la léproserie de la ville de Troyes,* Mémoires de la Société d'Agriculture, des Sciences, Arts et Belles-Lettres du Département de l'Aube, 2d series, I, nos. 7 and 8 (Troyes, 1848), 433.

marry; and that a leper could require a healthy wife to engage in sexual intercourse.[62] In the thirteenth century, Pope Gregory IX confirmed the Lateran decrees in a letter to Alexander III, the Archbishop of Canterbury. Gregory writes to the archbishop that it has come to his attention that healthy spouses do not remain with leprous husbands or wives who are separated from the community. Following the substance and intent of the council's decrees, Gregory states that leprosy is not a cause for the dissolution of marriage. To be sure, a leprous spouse has the right to demand that a healthy partner engage in sexual intercourse, though a husband and wife who do not wish to do so may abstain if each agrees to remain continent while the other is alive. If they refuse to observe these injunctions, they ought to be excommunicated. In short, "spouses must not be separated from marriage because of leprosy, and they [unmarried lepers] can contract a marriage, and are mutually bound to return the marriage debt to one another."[63] Thus, the Church maintained that leprosy could not essentially alter the nature of a marriage, and it did what it could to counter the natural tendency of a healthy man or woman to leave a diseased partner. The principles set forth by the Church had some effect upon marital practice. For instance, at certain places, such as Lisieux, "lepers were allowed not only to marry but to have servants and to live a family life."[64] In England also, where lepers were not inevitably regarded as dead by civil law, divorce as a result of leprosy was not inevitable; in fact, "statutory recogni-

---

[62] Jeanselme, p. 13.

[63] Gregorius IX, "De Coniugio leprosorum," *Decretales* (Basel, 1494), book IV, title VIII.

[64] Mercier, p. 15.

tion of leprosy as a cause for divorce in England" ended
with the Norman Conquest.[65] Nonetheless, Mercier states
that the usual situation was that the leper was declared dead
and the spouse was consequently free to remarry. Some
men, at least, took advantage of the opportunities made
available: "Lobineau, in his history of Britanny, says that
there were in the city of Dol several husbands who had
three wives living at the same time."[66] And at some places—
Reims, for example—it was decided not to celebrate a mass
over a leprous married woman at the ritual which separated her from society. The ceremony would point out to
to her that she is dead to the world, and her husband, taking the symbolic as literal, would find a new mate.[67]

In brief, the law could place a person outside of society
by depriving him of his rights to marry or to stay married,
and to own and transmit property. It could simply and
effectively deprive the leper of the right to have a home,
and that being so, it could compel him to depend upon the
very society which, out of loathing and fear, wrote those
laws. Under such circumstances, the best the leper could
do would be to turn from the world and enter the closed
society of the leprosarium. There, at least, he would have
a bed and food. The prison could also be a refuge.

Various kinds of evidence suggest that the leper house
could assume the character of a sanctuary. It has already
been pointed out that wealthy lepers would erect houses
on the grounds of leprosariums, and that some leprosariums
accepted only prosperous inmates. There are also records
of asylums which ultimately became places of retirement

[65] MacArthur "Some Notes," pp. 412–413.
[66] Mercier, p. 15.
[67] Cougoul, pp. 67 f.

rather than of segregation: for various reasons, healthy paying inmates were admitted along with the lepers who could not afford entry. The elderly would be permitted to enter the house in return for an annual fee or for willing all their wealth to the leprosarium.[68] The penalities imposed upon disobedient lepers afford additional evidence that the leprosarium could become a refuge. At the leper house of Greenside, Scotland, a leper who stayed outside the asylum for a night could be hung in punishment, but the house at St. Albans punished the same offense by expelling the leper from the house.[69] Though we are likely to think it no punishment at all to free a man, it is a punishment when the freedom brings greater hardship than confinement does. Accordingly, in many leper houses, severe infractions of the rules were punished with expulsion. In England's Sherburn Hospital, disobedient lepers were physically punished, as the prior or prioress saw fit, by being beaten like schoolchildren with a rod: "per ferulam modo scholiarium." Those especially difficult were fed on bread and water, but after the third offense, when they had proven they were past hope, they could be given the final punishment—banishment from the house.[70]

Direct testimony to the sanctuary leper houses could provide is given in poems written by Jean Bodel and Baude Fastoul when they were forced to leave their native city, Arras, and find asylum in leprosariums.[71] Bodel, the first of

---

[68] Delaunay, pp. 457 f. and Jeanselme, p. 83.

[69] Mercier, p. 16.

[70] Robert Surtees, *The History and Antiquities of the County Palatine of Durham*, I (London, 1816), 129. See also Le Grand, pp. 182, 185, 227, 243.

[71] "Les Congés de Jean Bodel," ed. Gaston Raynaud, *Romania*,

the pair to become a leper, wrote his "Congés" in 1202; Fastoul, who uses Bodel's poem as a model, wrote his fare-well and request for assistance sometime after Bodel's death (ca. 1210), for he seeks to obtain Bodel's place in a leper house: "je doi recevoir le fief /Ki vient de par Jehan Bodel" (227–228).

Written for similar reasons, the two "Congés" are alike in purpose and manner. In each case a man says goodby to his acquaintances and asks for help in obtaining entrance into a leprosarium, and in each case the hopelessness which forces him to plead for asylum is reflected in the pitiful leave-taking. Bodel is so sorrowful that his heart breaks, "si dolans que li cuers me crieve" (46); his sadness is with-out equal: "Me dolors totes autres passe" (259). The poet knows his disease cannot be cured. His own doctor has tried in vain:

> Coment osa il entreprendre
> Tel teste a roisnier et a fendre,
> Qui ert mauvaise tote entire?   [310–312]

(How did he dare undertake to shave and to fissure such a head, which was entirely diseased?)

And the combined efforts of all the physicians of Salerno would be equally without effect: "tuit li mire de Salerne / N'abaisseroient cheste lime" (201–202). Similarly, Fastoul writes of his own incurable disease, "Dont cascuns dist que nus ne sane" (170).

The desolation of the two men grows out of the cer-

IX (1880), 216–247. "Che sont li Congié Baude Fastoul d'Aras," in *Fabliaux et contes des poètes françois*, ed. Étienne Barbazan and M. Méon, I (Paris, 1808), 111–134. Quotations from the two poems are followed by line numbers, given in brackets or parentheses.

tainty of their deaths—and out of the other death each must face in life. Both must live isolated in a community of lepers, and it is of course that simple and overwhelming fact whch forces them to take their leave. Fastoul writes:

> Enfertés ki mon cors meshaigne,
> Pour coi tous li mons me desdaigne,
> Me fait de cascun estre eskiu.　　[301–303]

> (The disease which torments my body, for which society rejects me, causes everyone to avoid me.)

Bodel grieves that as a leper he can no longer eat with the healthy (94–96); the world will not let him cross his threshold (250); he has been cut off: "tos li mons me desacointe" (132).

The leper's physical suffering is compounded by the anguish of his exclusion from the world. He fears isolation as much as he fears death. For this reason, presumably, Bodel tried to conceal his disease, "L'enfretés que j'ai tant repuse" (151), but the leprosy could not be hidden indefinitely. Someone was bound to find him out. Bodel alludes to his exposure (245–246): "Refusé m'a et calengié / Li mons" (The world excluded me and prosecuted me).[72]

The trial which led to his expulsion must have been terrible for him, for he comments that it is better to leave freely than to be driven away (156). He states (343) that he lives

---

[72] Charles Foulon, *L'Oeuvre de Jehan Bodel* (Rennes, 1958), p. 737. Fastoul also seems to have undergone such an experience:

> Aler m'estuet en un desert,
> Puis que mi mal sont descouvert.　　[160–161]
> (It was necessary for me to go to a forsaken spot after my discomforts were discovered.)

on the outskirts of Arras ("Remés sui dedens le banliwe"), but apparently he cannot remain where he is for long, for he seeks aid in finding a permanent place at a leprosarium.[73]

Since entrance into an asylum usually required that the leper will his property to the house or make a payment to it, a man of small means often found it difficult to gain admission to one. In order to raise the needed funds Bodel appeals to the goodness of the mayor, Raol Ravuin, "gentius maire" (see 229–231):

> Se Deu plaist et se gentlelise,
> Ja en li ne perdrai men fief.   [473–474]

(If it is pleasing to God and to his [the mayor's] noblemen, through him [the mayor] I will not lose my fief [i.e., place, bed at a leprosarium].)

He also petitions the municipal magistrates, who ought to be moved by Bodel's plea, since he contracted the disease in their service (475–480):

> Seignor, ainchois que jo m'en aille,
> Vos proi a cheste definaille
> Por Deu et por nativite
> Qu'entre vos fachies une taille
> A parfornir cheste bataille
> Dort cascuns doit avoir pite.
> Mout m'aries bien airete.
> S'a Miaulens m'avies bote;
> Jo ne sai maison qui le vaille;
> Pieche a m'a li lius delite,
> Quar gent i a de carite:
> Bien me sofiroit lor vitaille.   [481–492]

---

[73] Foulon, pp. 731 f. Cf. Emile Langlade, *Jehan Bodel: Avec des commentaires sur le Congé de Baude Fastoul* (Paris, 1909), p. 257.

(Messeigneurs, before I leave you, I ask you at this crisis, in the name of God and our birthplace, that you get up a subscription among you to put an end to this difficulty, for which each one ought to have pity. You would have provided well for me if you had placed me in the leprosarium of Meulan; I do not know a house which could equal it; it is a place which has long pleased me, for charitable people are there: I should be well pleased with their sustenance.)

Similarly, when it became necessary for Fastoul to enter the leper colony, he turned to the town's administrators:

> Aler m'estuet à terme brief
> U je paierai grant relief
> Ains que j'aie pain ne tourtel,
> Eskievin on trouvé un brief
> Ke je doi recevoir le fief
> Ki vient de par Jehan Bodel.   [223–228]

(I have to go shortly to a place where I shall have to pay a large sum before I can have bread or cake. The scribes have found a document according to which I ought to receive the fief formerly held by Jean Bodel.)

The need of Bodel and Fastoul for asylum in the leper house emphasizes the harshness of life outside it. The poems suggest the abuse which the leper suffered, abuse which had its origin in the terror that the disease inspired in others. The leper was condemned, humiliated, and excluded. Bodel admits that he is "honteus" (62), shameful, just as Fastoul does when he writes that his disease makes him dejected and shameful: "Li maus . . . Me fait estre mas et honteus" (481, 483). The shame is of course a moral response to society's moral condemnation of leprosy, which both men accept. They understand that they are being punished by God. Bodel's God,

> Deus, qui tos biens acostumas,
> Qui de te verge batu m'as . . .   [353–354]

> (God, you who give all good, you who have beaten me with your ferule . . .)

is the same God who chastizes Fastoul:

> Cil Dix ki nului ne fait tort,
> Ki m'a batu devant le mort . . .   [532–533]

> (He, the God who wrongs no one, who has beaten me before death . . .)

The piety expressed by the two men may be not merely conventional, but deeply felt. The poets may well believe that all their suffering is for some greater end—Bodel, for example, anticipates that a life of poverty will purify his soul (237–240, 319–321)—but what emerges most forcefully, and with terrifying clarity, is the predicament of the leper in this world. He is a man who, although once a respected member of his society, has been cast out of it—and who must, in his forced isolation, plead with that society to purchase a bed for him in a leper house.

It is of course an irony of history that the very thing which made a leprosarium a place which could protect a leper from the world—that is, its wealth—could also convert it into the object of special oppression. Perhaps the most famous example of persecutions of leper houses is the action taken against them by Philip V (who ruled 1316–1322). Philip, whose coffers were ever in need of money, turned to the leper houses as sources of additional income.

By accusing lepers of having poisoned wells across France, but particularly in Languedoc, he succeeded in having hundreds of them burned to death, and the land and wealth of the leper houses appropriated for his own use.[74]

It is another curiosity of history that although lepers were the victims of constant persecution, abuse, and vilificaton, in general their mobility was not hampered and they were not effectively isolated from society. A mass of evidence suggests that in practice the sequestration of lepers was not rigidly enforced. The leper was not usually isolated unless mutilating and ulcerous lesions could be found.[75] Certain classes of lepers (for instance, the *cagots* of southern France, the so-called white lepers) lived more or less in freedom. For the most part, lepers were denied the usual legal privileges and protections, but although the *cagots* and others lived under severe regulations, they could own, sell, make contracts and wills, and under certain circumstances testify in court.[76] Furthermore, the leper houses did not succeed in totally isolating the lepers.[77] Even if lepers were forbidden to beg, they often could obtain permission to leave the house. For example, at the asylum at Rivery, they were permitted to leave every fifth day for Amiens, except during the summer, when contagion was

[74] Mercier, p. 17 and Ernest Wickersheimer, "Les Accusations d'empoisonnement portées pendant la première moitié du XIVe siècle contre les lépreux et les juifs; leurs relations avec les épidémies de peste," *Comptes-rendus du quatrième congrès international d'histoire de la médecine,* ed. Tricot-Royer and Laignel-Lavastine (Antwerp, 1927), pp. 76–83.

[75] Jeanselme, p. 60.

[76] Cougoul, p. 71.

[77] R. C. Holcomb, "The Antiquity of Congenital Syphilis," *Bull Hist Med,* X (1941), 150.

more feared than in winter. But there are evidences of
frequent infractions of even such a permissive rule.[78] In
any event, the French leper houses did not suffice to contain the ill, with the result that lepers circulated freely
across the countryside. Consequently, measures to restrict
their movement became increasingly severe, but they were
not always adhered to.[79] The situation was clearly similar
in England. Newman's study of English leprosariums shows
"that the general arrangements of the affairs of the leper
houses were in almost every way lax and irregular" (p. 31).
He cites a case concerning two supervisors of lepers who
were exempted from performing certain required obligations of their city, such as jury duty, because the necessity
to chastize lepers left them little time for other things.
Moreover, no leper could be made to enter an asylum if he
did not want to. He could choose to isolate himself in his
home, and the law could only be brought to bear against
him if he violated his seclusion—in which case he could be
forced into isolation by the writ *De Leproso Amovendo.*[80]
For instance, in 1372 the mayor and aldermen of London
ordered a baker named John Mayn to leave London "and
avoid the common conversation of mankind" because of his
leprosy. Mayn swore to leave and not return "on pain of
undergoing the punishment of the pillory."[81] A similar
writ was issued to force a certain J. de H. out of London:

The king [sends] greetings to the mayor and viscounts of

[78] Delaunay, p. 458.

[79] Cougoul, pp. 36–37. See also Jeanselme, pp. 3, 18, 112.

[80] MacArthur, "Medieval 'Leprosy' in the British Isles," p. 12,
and Newman, p. 31.

[81] *Memorials of London and London Life,* ed. and trans. Henry
Thomas Riley (London, 1868), pp. 365 f.

London. Because we have heard that J. de H. is a leper and
lives in the community with the men of the aforementioned
city, and has social intercourse with them in public places as
well as private, and refuses to move to a place of solitude as is
the custom and as it pertains to him, to the serious harm of the
above-mentioned men, and the danger is clear because of the
infectious nature of the above-mentioned disease: we, wishing
to guard against a danger of this sort as it pertains to us, and
wishing that what is just and customary be done for the sake of
the above-mentioned, we order you, taking aside with you some
prudent and unchallengeable men of the aforementioned city
who are not suspect, who have a rather good acquaintance
with the aforementioned J. and with disease of this sort, that
you approach J. himself and that you bring it about that he
be seen and examined diligently in the presence of the above-
mentioned men. And if you find him to be a leper as has been
said, then bring it about without delay that he be removed
from communication with the above-mentioned men in any
honorable way you can and have him move to a secluded place
for living there, as is the custom, so that no harm or danger
may come in some way to the aforementioned men through
common intercourse of this sort.[82]

MacArthur comments that the legal process involved in
obtaining and enforcing such as writ was too complicated
for it to be very effective: "Obviously such a cumbrous
and lengthy legal procedure could be undertaken in special
cases only, and the decree *De Leproso Amovendo* does not
appear to have been in general operation at any period."[83]

[82] *Registrum omnium breuiam tam originalium quam iudicialium*
(London, 1531), p. 267 and facing p. 268.
[83] MacArthur, "Some Notes on Old-Time Leprosy," p. 410. Cf.
Newman, p. 66: "The lepers were much shunned and lived much
in solitude,—but that there was in any sense a *strict* separation of

Public pronouncements, edicts, and laws emphasized that the leper was a doomed and dangerous man, a man to be avoided, isolated, shunned. If the laws were so severe that they could not be enforced, nevertheless they contributed to and publicized an attitude toward lepers expressed by Church fathers and physicians: in their physical corruption, lepers are morally corrupt. In 1346, Edward III issued a royal mandate excluding lepers from London:

Edward, by the grace of God, etc. Forasmuch as we have been given to understand that many persons, as well of the city aforesaid, as others coming to the said city, being smitten with the blemish of leprosy, do publicly dwell among the other citizens and sound persons, and there continually abide; and do not hesitate to communicate with them, as well in public places as in private; and that some of them, endeavouring to contaminate others with that abominable blemish, (that so, to their own wretched solace, they may have the more fellows in suffering), as well in the way of mutual communications, and by the contagion of their polluted breath, as by carnal intercourse with women in stews and other secret places, detestably frequenting the same, do so taint persons who are sound, both male and female, to the great injury of the people dwelling in the city aforesaid, and the manifest peril of other persons to the same city resorting;—We, wishing in every way to provide against the evils and perils which from the cause aforesaid may unto the said city, and the whole of our realm, arise, do command you, strictly enjoining, that, immediately on seeing these presents, you will cause it to be publicly proclaimed on our behalf in every Ward of the city aforesaid,

---

the diseased from the healthy, or that the *De Leproso Amovendo* was strictly and constantly enforced, I can find no substantial evidence. But I have found a very large mass of evidence to the contrary."

and in the suburbs thereof, where you shall deem it expedient, that all persons who have such blemish, shall, within fifteen days from the date of these presents, quit the City and the suburbs aforesaid, on the peril which is thereunto attached, and betake themselves to places in the country, solitary, and notably distant from the said city and suburbs, and take up their dwelling there; seeking their victuals, through such sound persons as may think proper to attend thereto, wheresoever they may deem it expedient. And that no persons shall permit such leprous people to dwell within their houses and buildings in the City, and in the suburbs aforesaid, on pain of forfeiture of their said houses and buildings, and more grievous punishment on them by us to be inflicted, if they shall contravene the same. And further, taking with you certain discreet and lawful men who have the best knowledge of this disease, all those persons, as well citizens as others, of whatever sex or condition they may be, whom, upon diligent examination in this behalf to be made, within the city and suburbs aforesaid you shall find to be smitten with the aforesaid blemish of leprosy, you are to cause to be removed from the communion of sound citizens and persons without delay, and taken to solitary places in the country, there, as above stated, to abide. And this, as you shall wish to keep yourselves scatheless, and to avoid our heavy indignation, you are not to delay doing; and as to that which you shall have done herein, you are distinctly and openly to certify us in our Chancery under your seals, within the fifteen days next ensuing herefrom. Witness myself, at Westminster, the 15th day of March, in the 20 year of our reign in England, and of our reign in France the 7th.[84]

The mandate makes clear that the disease is considered highly contagious (Edward fears that it will spread from

[84] *Memorials of London and London Life*, pp. 230–231.

the city through his realm), that numerous lepers come and go freely in the city, that some of the lepers seek solace through spreading the disease to others, and that they find satisfaction (and, it may be inferred, pleasure) in infecting others, particularly by "detestably frequenting" the houses of prostitutes "and other secret places." The threat is so great that Edward issues the equivalent of the writ *De Leproso Amovendo*, directing it to all lepers, without exception.

In 1375 Edward was once again called upon to restrict the lepers' mobility. The porters of the city gates were sworn to prevent lepers from entering the city. If a leper should attempt to enter in spite of a warning, his horse (if he had one) and outer garment were to be seized and held by the mayor at his discretion. If the leper should still try to pass, he was to be arrested and imprisoned for a length of time to be decided by the mayor. The lepers were clearly persistent and presumably successful, for the porters are warned that a failure to enforce the law could result in their being pilloried.[85]

The city of Paris also had its problems with lepers. In 1371 Charles V complained that lepers were roaming freely through the capital, infecting the healthy. He ordered those not born there or not permanently residing there to be expelled or incarcerated:

Il est venu à nostre congnoissance . . . que depuis le commencement de noz guerres, plusieurs hommes et femmes meseaux infectez de la maladie saint Ladre, . . . sont venus et viennent de jour en jour en nostre dite bonne Ville, en telle quantité et nombre, allans parmi la ville, querans leurs vies et aumosnes, buvans et mengens emmi les rües, ès carrefours et autres lieux publiques, où il passe le plus de gent, en telle

[85] *Memorials of London and London Life*, p. 384.

maniere qu'ilz empeschent et destourbent bien souvent les gens à passer ou à aller en leur besongnes que ilz passent parmi ou par empres eulz, et sentent leurs alaines, . . . par quoy nos bon subgez et populaires qui sont simples gens, pourroient par la compaignie et multitude des diz meseaulx aussi frequentants, alans et sejournans en nostre dite bonne Ville, estre infecs et ferus de la dite maladie saint Ladre.[86]

(It has come to our attention that since the outbreak of our wars [the Hundred Years War], many leprous men and women infected with the disease of Saint Ladre [i.e., Lazarus] . . . have come and are coming each day into our good city, in such quantity and number, going about the city, seeking their livelihood and alms, eating and drinking in the streets, squares, and other public places where many people pass—in such a manner that they frequently impede and divert the people from passing or from going about their business and that they pass among or alongside them, and smell their breath . . . by which our good subjects and commoners, who are simple people, may be infected and struck by the malady of Saint Ladre through the frequent company and multitude of lepers, moving about and residing in our good city.)

The provost of Paris issued similar decrees in 1388, 1394, 1402, and 1403. In 1404, Charles VI forbad entry of lepers into the city, and in 1413 forbad it at least once again. The constancy of incursions by lepers is suggested by the language of the edict of 1413, which is derived from decrees like the one issued in 1371 by Charles V:

. . . plusieurs hommes et femmes meseaulx et infects de la maladie de lepre, de jour en jour sont toujours allans et venans par lesdites Villes, querans leurs vies et aumosnes, bevans et mangeans parmy les rues, carrefours et autres lieux publiques

[86] Jeanselme, p. 18.

où il passe le plus de gens, en telle maniere qu'ils empeschent et destourbent bien souvent les gens à passer et aller en leurs besongnes, et faut qu'ils pasent parmy et emprès eux, et sentent leurs alaines qui est grand peril et puet tourner ou grand dommage de nos subgets.[87]

(. . . many leprous men and women, infected with the disease of leprosy, each day are constantly going and coming in the said city seeking their livelihood and alms, eating and drinking in the streets, squares and other public places where many people pass, in such a manner that they frequently impede and divert the people from passing or going about their business, and it is necessary that they pass among and alongside them, and smell their breath, which is a great danger and could result in great injury to our subjects.)

The Paris and London decrees illustrate common medieval attitudes toward the leper. In the frequency with which they were published, the edicts suggest not only the deep fear which leprosy could arouse, but also that the fear is not shared by all, that there are some, at least, who—like it or not—go through streets occupied by lepers, and even some with whom the lepers find shelter. The danger of leprosy is obviously not recognized by all the citizenry, for although Edward III complains that lepers spread their malady "to the great injury" and "manifest peril" of others, he must decree also that those harboring lepers do so "on pain of forfeiture of their said houses and buildings, and more grievous punishment on them by us to be inflicted." The world of the leper emerges as a world of contradiction and inconsistency—indeed, as a world which accomodated two incompatible ideas of leprosy: the disease was the sick-

[87] Jeanselme, pp. 18–21, 112.

ness both of the damned sinner and of one given special grace by God.

The idea of the leper as specially chosen by God for salvation was propagated primarily by the Church. The disease is early associated with divinity. For instance, St. Gregory of Nazianzus (ca. 325–390) writes, "We should above all be especially pitiful toward those afflicted with the Sacred Malady, who are gangrenous and rotten of flesh, even to their bones and the marrow of their bones."[88] In 1239, the bishop of Tournai urged that the disease is a gift from God.[89] The Parson in the *Canterbury Tales* injects a similar idea while speaking of the evils of chiding and reproach:

And taak kep now, that he that repreveth his neighebor, outher he repreveth hym by som harm of peyne that he hath on his body, as "mesel," "croked harlot," or by som synne that he dooth. Now if he repreve hym by harm of peyne, thanne turneth the repreve to Jhesu Crist, for peyne is sent by the rightwys sonde of God, and by his suffrance, be it meselrie, or mayheym, or maladie.[90]

(And take heed now, that he who reproves his neighbor, finds fault either with some affliction that he has on his body, as by calling him "leper," "crooked rascal," or with some sin that he does. Now if he reproves him for some affliction, then the reproof turns against Jesus Christ, for affliction is sent by the righteous sending of God, and with his permission, be it leprosy, or mayhem, or disease.)

[88] Brown, p. 299. For the original, see "Oratio XIV: De pauperum amore," 261 (*PG*, XXXV, 866).

[89] Delaunay, p. 457.

[90] Geoffrey Chaucer, ParsT, 624–625, in *The Works of Geoffrey Chaucer*, ed. F. N. Robinson, 2d ed. (Boston, 1957).

The idea of leprosy as a disease inflicted by God, usually offered as a comfort to lepers, found justification in the Bible, where Lazarus is the model of the chosen leper. Luke retells the parable of the beggar, "full of sores," who asks to be fed with crumbs which fell from a rich man's table.

And it came to pass, that the beggar died, and was carried by the angels into Abraham's bosom. And the rich man also died: and he was buried in hell. And lifting up his eyes when he was in torments, he saw Abraham afar off, and Lazarus in his bosom: And he cried and said: Father Abraham, have mercy on me, and send Lazarus, that he may dip the tip of his finger in water, to cool my tongue, for I am tormented in this flame. And Abraham said to him: Son, remember that thou didst receive good things in thy lifetime, and likewise Lazarus evil things, but now he is comforted; and thou art tormented.

[16:22–25]

According to a Latin chronicler, Louis VII (ca. 1120–1180) spoke to lepers of Lazarus "in order that they—burdened by infirmity of body—will study to deserve the health of their souls."[91] The parable is also alluded to in the ritual of separation used in the diocese of Vienne. The priest speaks to the leper who is about to be sequestered:

My friend, it pleases our Lord that you should be infected with this disease, and our Lord gives you a great gift when He wishes to punish you for the evil you have done in this world. Wherefore have patience in your illness, for our Lord does not spurn you because of your disease, nor separate you from His company. But if you have patience you shall be saved, as was the leper who died before the house of Dives, and was taken directly into paradise.[92]

[91] Delaunay, p. 457.
[92] J. A. Ulysse Chevalier, *Notice historique sur la maladrerie de Voley près Romans* (Romans, 1870), p. 34.

Guy of Chaulic instructs physicians to give similar comfort to lepers during the diagnosis:

In the first place, invoking the aid of God, he ought to comfort them by saying that this illness is the salvation of the soul, and that they ought not at all to fear to say the truth: for if they are found lepers, that will be the purgatory of their soul, and if the world loathes them, God—who loved the leprous Lazarus more than others—does not.[93]

These assurances clearly offered to lepers an antidote for the prevailing view that leprosy was a sure sign of inner moral decay. Following the First Crusade, when soldiers returned to Europe infected with leprosy, there was particular need for Christians to disassociate leprosy and sin, for Peter the Hermit had promised absolution from sin and ultimate salvation to those who fought the holy war, and now the army was returning, carrying with it the disease which according to some marked men as sinners. The difficulty was reconciled through recourse to passages such as the parable of Lazarus and especially through an interpretation of Isaiah 53:4:

Vere languores nostros ipse tulit et dolores nostros ipse portavit, et nos putavimus eum quasi leprosum et percussam a Deo et humiliatum.

(Surely he hath borne our infirmities and carried our sorrows: and we have thought him as it were a leper, and as one struck by God and afflicted.)

The passage was taken as a prophesy concerning Jesus. If we read *leprosum* traditionally, the verse suggests only that Jesus would be "stricken." However, if we take the word literally, the verse tells that Jesus would be "esteemed

[93] *La Grande Chirvrgie*, p. 405. See also Jeanselme, p. 50.

leprous." In this way, leprosy indeed comes to be viewed as a sacred malady.[94] The association of the disease with Jesus is seen in numerous sermons. The preachers told stories of how Jesus would appear before the faithful in the form of a leper. In one such story, a monk named Martyrius comes upon a leper who cannot walk. The monk carries the leper to the monastery; as Martyrius approaches the monastery, the abbot sees that his monk is carrying Christ.[95] Another tale tells how a certain pious Count Theobald cared for a leper who lived in a hut outside the village of Sezenna. Unknown to Theobald, the leper died; however, when the count went to the hut to visit the leper, he found him in the hut as usual. Later, after learning that the leper had been dead for some time, the count returned to the hut and was greeted by an odor of sweetness—a sign given by the Lord to show how pleasing he considers works of piety.[96] These and other *exempla* of the sort were a regular part of the preachers' collections of moral anecdotes.[97]

The older notion of leprosy as the sinner's disease prevailed, however, in spite of all the pious commentary and preaching to the contrary. Even in the Vienne ritual, the

[94] Feeny, pp. 25, 31–32. See also MacArthur, "Medieval 'Leprosy,'" p. 11.

[95] *The Homilies of the Anglo-Saxon Church: The First Part, Containing the Sermones Catholici, or Homilies of Aelfric*, ed. and trans. Benjamin Thorpe, I (London, 1844), 337.

[96] Sermon XCIV, *The Exempla or Illustrative Stories from the Sermones Vulgares of Jacques de Vitry*, ed. Thomas Frederick Crane, Publications of the Folk-Lore Society, XXVI (London, 1890), 43–44; Caesarius of Heisterbach, *The Dialogue on Miracles*, trans. H von E. Scott and C. C. Swinton Bland, II (London, 1929), 30–31.

[97] See Sermon XCV, *The Exempla of Jacques de Vitry*, pp. 44–45; *The Dialogue on Miracles*, II, 31–34.

priest is constrained to say that the disease is a punishment "for the evil you have done in this world." In his sermon asking compassion for lepers, Gregory of Nazianzus calls them "men already dead except to sin." At St. Alban's, the lepers are reminded "to bear themselves as more to be despised and as more humble than all other men." Rothar permits a man to break his engagement to a woman who becomes leprous through sin. And of course it was the lepers' reputation for evil which enabled Philip V to turn the population of France against them. Thus, although society's attitude toward lepers was ambivalent, the notion that they were morally depraved produced effects more immediate and more enduring than those produced by the promise of divine grace. While the leper might look forward to salvation after death, his experience in life could not help but taint his mind. Theodoric the physician describes the leper as wrathful, malevolent, and mistrustful—he suspects everyone wants to hurt him.[98] Though a comment such as Theodoric's may seem to describe an unreasonable perversity, behind the leper's suspicion lies an understandable response to the world. Society organized itself against the leper. When it discovered his presence, he was excluded, often by means of the grim ritual which forced him to stand in a grave while mass was said over him. Declared dead to the world, he might be banished to a leper house or simply banished, forced to rely on the mercy of a world which feared and abused him. Disowned by society, he would move from town to town as one of the many beggars mayors were

[98] *The Surgery of Theodoric*, trans. Eldridge Campbell and James Colton, II (New York, 1960), 171.

called upon to exclude. And underlying all of it—beneath ecclesiastical edicts, medical diagnoses, legal decisions, municipal decrees—was the almost ubiquitous assumption that his leprosy was a punishment for sin.

III

The Ecclesiastical Tradition

"What strange ideas people have about leprosy, doctor."
"They learn it from the Bible. Like sex."
                    Graham Greene, *A Burnt-Out Case*

Leprosy in the Middle Ages was a disease of the soul as well as the body, and although the leper carried many burdens, few were so heavy as his reputation for immorality. He contracted his reputation along with his disease, for the stigma inevitably followed the illness. The association of leprosy and sinfulness was as persistent as the disease itself.

To locate the source of the leprosy stigma in the Bible is tempting—but the Bible merely contains evidence of the stigma, not of its origin. The connection between leprosy and immorality was established before the Bible was written, and it has appeared nearly everywhere the disease has. The moral associations of leprosy are not the exclusive property of the Bible, nor are they even confined to Western culture. For example, Chinese attitudes toward leprosy have been shown to be comparable to European attitudes such as those expressed in the Bible, and independent of them.[1] Further, it seems inescapable that what the Bible

---

[1] Olaf K. Skinsnes, "Leprosy in Society: 'Leprosy Has Appeared on the Face,'" *Leprosy Rev*, XXXV (1964), 35.

does say is not being said for the first time; rather, the Bible preserves, codifies, and elaborates tradition.[2] However, none of these assertions casts doubt on the influence of the Bible, for even if it is not the source of the leper's reputation for sinfulness, no other document can claim to have helped so much in propagating that reputation.

Lepers and leprosy make frequent appearances in the Bible. Explicit mention of them occurs in Exodus, Numbers, Deuteronomy, in II Samuel, II Kings, and II Chronicles, and in Matthew, Mark, and Luke. But it is the Book of Leviticus that contains the most detailed and extended description of leprosy in the Bible. Leviticus, a compilation of laws, gives minute instructions concerning sacrificial ritual, the installation of priests, cleanness and uncleanness, the observance of the Day of Atonement, and other ceremonies and obligations. Of the book's twenty-seven chapters, two are given over to the discussion of leprosy, a discussion which can be understood only if examined in relation to the rest of Leviticus.

Two of the key words in Leviticus are *tahor*, clean, and *tameh*, unclean. They describe opposed conditions, conditions of purity and impurity, holiness and unholiness. If something is clean, it is undefiled and therefore pleasing to God, since it duplicates the purity of God:

For I the Lord am your God: you shall sanctify yourselves and be holy, for I am holy. You shall not make yourselves unclean through any swarming thing that moves upon the earth.

[2] Roland de Vaux, *Ancient Israel: Its Life and Institutions*, trans. John McHugh (New York, 1961), pp. 460, 463–464. Yehezkel Kaufmann, *The Religion of Israel: From Its Beginnings to the Babylonian Exile*, trans. Moshe Greenberg (Chicago, 1960), pp. 447–448.

For I the Lord am He who brought you up from the land of Egypt to be your God. You shall be holy, for I am holy.[3]

In Leviticus, both holiness and cleanness are connected with religious ritual, and the book's regulations are in large part instructions intended to insure that the sanctified enclosure—the Tabernacle or Tent of Meeting[4]—not be defiled: "You shall put the Israelites on guard against their uncleanness, lest they die through their uncleanness by defiling My Tabernacle which is among them."[5] Thus, Leviticus defines what would defile a place of worship or would keep a worshiper from entering into it.

For instance, chapter 11 distinguishes clean and unclean creatures, those which may be eaten and those which may not. Land animals without cloven hoofs or which do not chew cud—camels, hares, and swine, among others—are un-

---

[3] Leviticus 11:44–45. Quotations from the Pentateuch are taken from *The Torah: The Five Books of Moses,* trans. Harry M. Orlinsky et al. (Philadelphia, 1962). For the criteria used in selecting editions and translations of the Bible, see Chapter II, n. 2.

[4] Classical biblical criticism urges that the Levitical Tabernacle is not any place of worship but only the Jerusalem Temple, "the site that the Lord your God will choose amidst all your tribes as His habitation, to establish His name there" (Deuteronomy 12:5). This conclusion is based upon the belief that Leviticus was written after Deuteronomy, and at a time when worship was centralized at the Temple. However, the classical dating has recently been shaken, and it no longer appears necessary to assume that "Tabernacle" was a metaphor for "Jerusalem Temple." Accordingly, Leviticus is no longer taken to have been written with the intention of dictating priestly practices in the Temple. Rather, it is now thought that although the legislation later became applicable in the Temple, it originally guided observances in "many legitimate local sanctuaries, each of which is represented here by the tent." See Kaufmann, p. 153 et passim, pp. 180–187.

[5] Leviticus 15:31. See also 22:9. Cf. Numbers 5:1–4.

clean, as are water creatures which do not have fins and
scales. Certain birds; all winged, swarming creatures that
walk on fours and lack jointed legs; and lizards, moles, and
mice are also unclean. In the same category are a woman
following sexual intercourse or childbirth, or during men-
struation (chap. 12 and 15:19–27), and a man with "a
discharge issuing from his member," or after an emission of
semen, or after sexual intercourse (chap. 12). So too is the
leper unclean, and cloth or skins or a house marked by what
is called leprosy (chaps. 13–14).

Hence, two varieties of uncleanness are named—uncleanness of things and human uncleanness. What is common to
both unclean types is that they are not holy, that is, not fit
to be associated with observances in the sanctuary. It is
important to recognize that uncleanness in Leviticus does
not imply moral guilt: a camel is not sinful, nor is a mouse,
nor a new mother, nor a house with reddish streaks, nor a
leper. The implications of uncleanness are ritualistic and
cultic, not ethical. Aside from the fact that he could not
enter a sanctuary or eat consecrated foods, "the worth and
status of an unclean person differed in no way from that of
a clean person":

> In themselves the alternatives *clean* and *unclean* involve no
> element of legal, moral, or religious valuation or violation; they
> bespeak neither merit nor demerit, neither virtue nor guilt, and
> apply to inanimate objects . . . no less than to men.[6]

Whether or not the Hebrews elsewhere attached moral implications to leprosy, in the Book of Leviticus those over-

---

[6] Julian Obermann, ed., *The Code of Maimonides: Book Ten,
The Book of Cleanness*, trans. Herbert Danby, Yale Judaica Series, VIII (New Haven, 1954), viii.

tones are missing. The leper may be unclean, and in order to purify himself he may have to make an offering and have the priest make expiation for him (see Leviticus 14:1–32), but nowhere does Leviticus state that leprosy is caused by sin. Rather, leprosy causes a man to be impure, a state defined as "an absence of holiness, an estrangement from YHWH [i.e., Yaweh, God], the source of all holiness. . . . Impurity is no more than a condition—one might almost say a religious-aesthetic state."[7] In any condition of impurity, a man is denied the privileges of normal life. The leper, for instance, is sent to an impure place outside the camp or city until such time as a priest can declare him clean. His isolation is demanded because his uncleanness is contagious, and uncleanness must not defile the holy sanctuary in the camp. That the leper's impurity is cultic rather than moral is revealed by the procedures given for cleansing the leper. Nowhere in the rituals are moral values put into play.

Time, ritual, and sacrifice remove impurity. The leper must remain outside the city for at least seven days before he can be declared ready for purification by a priest. When the leper is found to be free of his leprosy, the priest begins the ritual of purification. First the pollution is transferred to a bird which is carried outside the camp and then released. Seven days later, the leper shaves himself and washes his body and clothing. On the eighth day, he brings unblemished lambs, a mixture of choice flour and oil, and a measure of oil to "be presented before the Lord, with the man to be cleansed, at the entrance of the Tent of Meeting, by the priest who performs the cleansing" (Leviticus

[7] Kaufmann, pp. 127, 103. See also de Vaux, p. 460.

14:11). The lambs, flour, and oil are used in making various offerings to God, including what are termed guilt and sin offerings, to obtain "expiation for the one being cleansed of his uncleanness" (14:19), the same kind of uncleanness which attached to a woman after childbirth.[8]

The cultic nature of the leprosy ritual is made plain by the fact that the priest's function is not to collect a debt owed to society, but to purify and "to make expiation before the Lord for the one being cleansed" (14:31). The expiation itself is not for a moral outrage, but must be made because a taboo has been broken. The offense of being a leper is not a willful act but is accidental, and the violation is not of human but of divine law. Consequently, the leper must appease God, make atonement to Him, just as a man must for a house tainted by leprosy (14:33–53). He is neither guilty nor innocent but simply unclean, unfit to enter a place consecrated to God.

In short, the Book of Leviticus does not judge the leper; it merely defines him as one of the group of persons and things ritually impure. Yet the terms for moral valuation— terms such as guilt, sin, and expiation—are all in the text. For the moral connotations to gather around Levitical leprosy, all that was needed was for the cultic context to be weakened, and two grounds for that weakening exist in the Old Testament itself. First, Leviticus does not deny that leprosy is a punishment for sin; it simply ignores the idea. Second, other parts of the Old Testament make the

[8] On guilt and sin offerings, see Kaufmann, pp. 112–115. Cf. de Vaux, *Ancient Israel*, pp. 418–421, 460–464, and *Studies in Old Testament Sacrifice* (Cardiff, 1964), pp. 91–95, 98–102. De Vaux comments that it is neither possible to distinguish the two offerings clearly nor "to state clearly the moral aspect of the sin which is expiated by these sacrifices" (*Ancient Israel*, p. 421).

connection between leprosy and sin explicit. Accordingly, it was natural that biblical commentators would come to the conclusion that the leprous uncleanness described in Leviticus was a consequence of the sins mentioned in stories such as the one about Miriam, for example.[9]

Miriam and Aaron, Moses' brother and sister, rebuke Moses because he marries a Cushite woman, a woman not even an Israelite, who presumably comes to share her husband's prestige. Their envy of Moses' wife leads them to assert that they are the equals of Moses. God, hearing them, rebukes them for speaking against their brother and causes Miriam to be covered with snow-white scales, the leprous affliction described in Leviticus 13:2–3. Aaron, seeing immediately that the leprosy is a punishment for their sin, turns to Moses, saying, "O my lord, account not to us the sin which we committed in our folly" (Numbers 12:11).

Leprosy also comes as a punishment when Uzziah, one of the kings of Judah, usurps the role of a priest by burning incense in the temple of the Lord.[10] When the priests try to stop him, he grows angry, but

a lesion broke out on the skin of his forehead before the priests

[9] Of course, Christian commentators had an additional reason for linking leprosy and sin. When the Hebrew came to be translated into Greek and then Latin, the words used to translate *tameh* ("unclean") were the Greek *akathartos* and the Latin *immundus*, words which in the Middle Ages had no cultic sense, but which did have distinct moral connotations. See Walter Bauer, *A Greek-English Lexicon of the New Testament and other Early Christian Literature*, trans. William F. Arndt and F. Wilbur Gingrich, 4th ed. (Chicago, 1957), p. 28; Albert Blaise, *Dictionnaire Latin-Française des auteurs Chrétiens* (Turnhout, Belgium, 1954), p. 409.

[10] See II Chronicles 26:16–23. Cf. II Kings 15:1–6, where the king is called Azariah and is punished by God with leprosy for failing to remove local sanctuaries.

in the house of Yaweh . . . [and] behold leprosy was on his forehead and they hurried him out of there; and he also was anxious to get out because Yaweh had afflicted him. Uzziah the king was thus a leper to the day of his death and lived in house of quarantine as a leper because he was excluded from the house of Yaweh.[11]

A third instance of leprosy as a divinely inflicted punishment for sin occurs in the Second Book of Kings, where Gehazi is striken with the disease by Elisha, "the man of God,"[12] as a chastisement for covetousness (5:20–27). The Old Testament, then, contains at least three instances where the connection between leprosy and a moral violation is explicit, and in each of the instances, the disease comes from God.

Among the earliest of the Hebrew commentaries on passages such as these is the *Midrash Rabbah*, a collection of interpretations of the Old Testament begun in the second century A.D. The views expressed in the Midrash are by no means consistent—rather, the book is a collection of varying interpretations of the biblical text; but if the writers who deal with leprosy do not necessarily agree on what sin or sins cause leprosy, there is at least no question that it is a sinner's disease. For instance, in a discussion of Deuteronomy 24:9 ("Remember what the Lord your God did to Miriam on the journey after you left Egypt"), the problem of why leprosy comes is raised. One view is that the disease is a punishment for grudging selfishness, but a second opinion maintains:

[11] 26:19, 20–21 in *II Chronicles*, trans. Jacob M. Myers, The Anchor Bible, vol. XIII (Garden City, N.Y., 1965).

[12] On the relationship between God and the Man of God, see Kaufmann, p. 85: "By God's will he reveals hidden things, works wonders, heals, blesses, and curses."

Plagues [of leprosy] come on account of nought save slander. The Rabbis say: A proof that the plagues come on account of slander can be derived from the case of the pious Miriam. Because she uttered slander against her brother Moses, plagues attacked her.[13]

Elsewhere the exegetes take a broader view of the moral causes of leprosy than the passages from the commentary on Deuteronomy do. For instance, the commentary on Leviticus 14:2 contains a list of seven sins which bring leprosy,[14] the seven things which are given as an abomination to God in Proverbs 6:17–19:

> Proud eyes, a lying tongue,
> Hands that shed the blood of the innocent,
> A mind full of evil schemes,
> Feet running toward wrong;
> A false witness breathing out lies,
> And one who stirs up quarrels between brothers.[15]

Elsewhere, a list of ten sins is given:

(i) idol-worship, (ii) gross unchastity [i.e., incest and adultery], (iii) bloodshed, (iv) the profanation of the Divine Name, (v) blasphemy of the Divine Name, (vi) robbing the public, (vii) usurping a dignity to which one has no right, (viii) overweening pride, (ix) evil speech [i.e., calumny, scan-

[13] "Deuteronomy," trans. J. Rabbinowitz, pp. 125–126 in *Midrash Rabbah*, ed. H. Freedman and Maurice Simon (London, 1939), VII. This opinion became traditional in Jewish commentary. See Moses Maimonides, *The Guide for the Perplexed* (ca. 1190), trans. M. Friedländer, 4th ed. (New York, 1927), pp. 369 f.: "All [our sages] agree that leprosy is a punishment for slander."

[14] "Leviticus," trans. J. Israelstam and Judah Slotki, in *Midrash Rabbah*, IV, 199.

[15] *Proverbs, Ecclesiastes,* trans. R. B. Y. Scott, The Anchor Bible, vol. XVIII (Garden City, N.Y., 1965).

dal], and (x) an evil eye [i.e., greediness, a grudging disposition].[16]

In order to prove that the sins named are sources of leprosy, the commentators point to biblical passages which connect, or seem to connect, leprosy and particular sins. The case of Miriam shows that evil speech or a lying tongue causes leprosy. Gehazi's disease shows that leprosy comes from profanation of the Divine Name or from feet that are swift in running to evil. Uzziah's instance connects leprosy with the sin of wicked thoughts in one list, and with two sins in the other—usurping an undeserved dignity and overweening pride. That haughty eyes are punished with leprosy is proved through the haughty daughters of Zion (Isaiah 3:16–17), whom the Lord will smite with a scab; in the second list, the same daughters establish that leprosy punishes unchastity. One of the exegetes presents the experience of Goliath as evidence that blaspheming the Divine Name produces leprosy. Goliath, who "cursed David by his god" (I Samuel 17:43), is proved to have been smitten with leprosy, since the verb used by David when he says, "This day will the Lord deliver (*sagar*) thee into my hand" (17:46) is the same verb used in discussing leprosy in Leviticus 13:5 and elsewhere: "the priest shall isolate (*sagar*) the leper."

Thus, the Midrashic commentators use the Bible to show that leprosy is a punishment for wickedness and, where the Bible is vague or inconclusive, they seek to uncover precisely what sins are punished by leprosy. Their different interpretations lead them to accumulate veritable catalogues of moral violations.

[16] "Leviticus," *Midrash Rabbah*, IV, 215.

In addition, the writers of Midrashim include popular tales, legends, and myths in their discussions of the Scripture. According to one such legend, before God presented the Law to His people, he sent angels to remove all diseases and afflictions from them, since he did not want "a race of cripples" to receive the Torah. However, when the Hebrews later defected from God and worshiped the Golden Calf, "all their diseases returned as a punishment for their defection from God." Still later, after the erection of the Tabernacle, God separated the unclean and the lepers from the camp, in order that they not defile it:

The law in regard to lepers was particularly severe, for they were denied the right of staying within the camp, whereas the unclean were prohibited merely from staying near the sanctuary. The lepers were the very ones who had worshipped the Golden Calf, and had as a consequence been smitten with this disease, and it was for this reason that God separated them from the community.[17]

Another legend deals with the story of Abram and Sarai in Egypt (Genesis 12:1–20). Abram instructs Sarai to say that she is his sister, not his wife, so that the Egyptians will not kill him in order to take her. When they arrive in Egypt, Pharoah takes Sarai for his own and presents Abram with magnificent gifts. According to the legend, Pharoah brings the woman into the royal bed chamber, but at each of his attempts to lead Sarai to bed, an angel sent by God strikes him a blow. And in the morning, leprosy appears "on the walls, beams and pillars of his bed chamber, and on the faces of his eunuchs." Sarai then confesses that she is mar-

---

[17] Louis Ginzberg, *The Legends of the Jews*, trans. Henrietta Szold and Paul Radin, III (Philadelphia, 1911), 212–213.

ried to Abram, and Pharaoh—recognizing the wrong he
nearly did—returns Sarai to her husband along with gifts
more magnificent than those first given. "Thereupon the
leprosy faded."[18] The moral of the story is clear, though
unwritten: adultery is a sin, and God's anger will fall upon
the man who commits adultery. The leprosy is sent by
God as a warning to Pharoah, and removed when the
warning is heeded. In sum, Midrashic commentary identifies leprosy as a punishment for sin. It spells out leprosy's
moral context, and that context becomes traditional in
Hebrew exegesis.

The commentary on Leviticus found in the *Mikra'oth
Gedoloth*—a book containing versions of the Old Testament in Hebrew and Aramaic, with accompanying glosses
—is a collection of the opinions of venerable Jewish exegetes. Three passages on the leprosy law—from writers
active during the thirteenth, seventeenth, and eighteenth
centuries—clearly draw upon Midrashic interpretations
and thus attest to the enduring strength of tradition in shaping attitudes toward leprosy. Orchaim (1696–1747) confirms the Midrashic notion that leprosy is a punishment for
spreading evil tales about a person; to the sin of slander,
Klai Yakar (d. 1619) adds two causes of leprosy—grossness
of spirit and a leering eye—at the same time noting that a
list of seven sins is to be found in the Talmud, and one of
ten in the Midrash. He emphasizes the rabbinical tradition
that sees leprosy as an external manifestation of spiritual
evil and a punishment of the evil. The fact that there is no

[18] Robert Graves and Raphael Patai, *Hebrew Myths: The Book
of Genesis* (New York, 1964), p. 144. The story is taken from
Midrashim dating from the fourth, eighth or ninth, and twelfth
centuries.

known natural cure for leprosy (doctors, he notes, have despaired of discovering one) indicates its divine origin and suggests that it can be alleviated only by moral regeneration. Similarly, Nahmanides (1195–ca. 1270) interprets leprosy, especially of houses or garments, as the external revelation of internal evil: when Israel is pure and faithful to God, he writes, then God's holy spirit hovers over the people and gives them and their possessions a favorable appearance. When one sins, however, the resultant ugliness of the leprosy which defiles his clothes or house or body is a sign that God has removed His holy spirit from that man.[19]

The study of attitudes toward leprosy within the Jewish tradition demonstrates that, by the medieval period, the idea of leprosy as a consequence of sin was firmly established. How much of medieval Christendom's view of leprosy is derived from Jewish culture is difficult to determine, however. To the degree that Jewish and Christian attitudes are European, and to the degree that both are products of Mediterranean culture, there are analogous and even identical ideas. For instance, the rabbis' statement that if a woman has sexual intercourse during her menstrual period she will produce a leprous child,[20] is a commonplace among medieval Christian writers, such as Bartholomeus Anglicus.[21] It is very unlikely that these writers or their authori-

---

[19] "Sefer Wayikra," *Mikra'oth Gedoloth* (New York, 1959), III, 146–147, 169, 161.

[20] "Leviticus," *Midrash Rabbah*, IV, 193.

[21] See Chapter I. See also two translations of Friar Lorens' *Somme des Vices et Vertus* (1279): *Dan Michel's Ayenbite of Inwit* (1340), ed. Richard Morris, EETS, No. 23 (London, 1866), pp. 223–224; *The Book of Vices and Virtues: A Fourteenth Cen-*

ties made a study of the Midrash; in all probability, the
rabbis and the Christians were merely articulating an idea
which was part of the current stock of popular knowledge.
Nonetheless, Jewish thought undoubtedly had some direct
influence on medieval Christian attitudes toward leprosy,
not only in Spain, where Jewish intellectuals were able to
establish themselves as physicians, translators, financiers,
and advisors to Christians, but also elsewhere.[22] This is not
to suggest significant direct contact between Hebrew and
Christian biblical scholars, however, for the commentaries
written by them were prepared independently for the most
part. Yet if their understandings are analogous, it is not
surprising, since both groups were involved in the study
of the same document, the Old Testament, a book which

---

*tury English Translation of the "Somme le Roi" of Lorens d'Or-
léans*, ed. W. Nelson Francis, EETS, O.S., no. 217 (London,
1942), p. 248.

[22] See Beryl Smalley, *The Study of the Bible in the Middle
Ages*, 2d ed. (Oxford, 1952), p. xvi: "A desire to study the text of
the Old Testament would always lead scholars to compare the
Latin with the Hebrew. The study of the Hebrew would always
lead to contact with Jews. The Christians lacked an unbroken
tradition of skill in semitic languages which would have enabled
them to dispense with Jewish help, had they wished to do so. In
fact, far from avoiding the Jews, Latin scholars asked them for
information on rabbinics as well as for guidance in the Hebrew
tongue. The Jews of northern France and the Rhineland, from
Rashi onward, supplemented their traditional lore by an original
method of exegesis. Hence Christians of the twelfth and thirteenth
centuries who consulted the rabbis would get two types of answer
to their questions: they would collect old traditions and specimens
of the traditional interpretation, and they would make the acquaintance of a living contemporary scholarship, which could
influence their own approach." Smalley provides the particular
instance of Andrew of St. Victor, who was familiar with Jewish
exegetes and substantially influenced by them (see pp. 149–172).

identifies leprosy as a divinely inflicted punishment. In brief, a reading of Christian biblical commentary indicates that the ecclesiastical authors received the notion that leprosy is the sinner's disease primarily from their culture, from the Old Testament, and from each other, not from the Hebrew exegetes. Like the rabbis, they connect leprosy and spiritual defilement, but they approach the Bible very differently.

For Christians, the Hebrew Scriptures were the Old Testament, the old law, the law revealed to the Jews by God but now superseded by the gospels. The Epistle to the Hebrews told Christians that the new convenant "hath made the former old. And that which decayeth and groweth old, is near its end" (8:13). Nonetheless, Christians did not allow the Old Testament to be discarded, for Jesus was the Christ, the Messiah who fulfilled Old Testament prophecy: "Do not think that I am come to destroy the law, or the prophets. I am not come to destroy, but to fulfil" (Matthew 5:17). The Old Testament was accepted as divinely inspired prophetic truth, and the interpretation of it therefore aimed at showing how the events and things contained in it prefigured the Christian fulfillment of history. St. Paul uses this approach to the Old Testament in his Epistles. In I Corinthians 10, he comments upon certain passages in Exodus and Numbers in order to reveal how the Old Testament events hold significance for Christians:

For I would not have you ignorant, brethren, that our fathers were all under the cloud, and all passed through the sea. And all in Moses were baptized, in the cloud and in the sea: And did all eat the same spiritual food, And all drank the same spiritual drink; (and they drank of the spiritual rock that followed them, and the rock was Christ.) But with most of them God was not well pleased: for they were overthrown in the desert. Now these things were done in a figure of us, that we should not covet evil things as they also coveted.   [vv. 1–6]

By studying the Old Testament, Paul was able to produce spiritual insights and moral lessons for Christians; here, he counsels them to avoid idolatry, fornication, tempting Christ, and murmuring. The acts of the Hebrews illustrate these sins, and they are recorded in the Bible for the purpose of teaching Christians to shun them. "Now all these things happened to them in figure: and they are written for our correction, upon whom the ends of the world are come" (v. 11). Through this technique, Paul elaborated a series of allegorical interpretations and figurative concepts—and by his example, he stimulated other commentators to read the Bible so as to unveil its spiritual significance.

The interpretation of the Scripture uncovered spiritual meanings of more than one kind. Indeed, some commentators found as many as seven levels of meaning, although most recognized four.[23] First was of course the literal meaning of the text, that is, the strict meaning of the words as opposed to spiritual meanings[24]—for instance, the healing of Naaman the leper in the Jordan river construed as a real immersion which cleansed a physical condition. Second was the allegorical level, on which the Old Testament fore-

---

[23] See the studies of medieval exegesis by Henri de Lubac, *Exégèse médiévale: Les quatres sens de l'Écriture*, 2 vols. (Paris, 1959–1964); Beryl Smalley, *The Study of the Bible in the Middle Ages*; and C[eslaus] Spicq, *Esquisse d'une histoire de l'exégèse latine au moyen âge*, Bibliothèque Thomiste, vol. XXVI (Paris, 1944).

[24] On the philosophical relationships between the literal and spiritual levels, see Anthony Nemetz, "Literalness and the *Sensus Litteralis*," *Spec*, XXXIV (1959), 76–89.

shadowed the New, or on which either Testament might refer to the Church (Naaman's healing interpreted as a prefiguration of Christ's baptism). The tropological sense was the third; it had reference to the moral state of the individual (Naaman's immersion taken as a reference to the need to cleanse one's soul). At the fourth level, the anagogical, which dealt with heaven and the afterlife, Naaman's entry into the water might be understood as the movement of the soul from this life to the next.

Thus, through the exegesis of the Old Testament, the commentators extracted anticipations of the life of Jesus, of religious practices and doctrines, and of Church history. The patristic use of allegory to harmonize the Old and New Testaments produced results which, in the words of Caesarius of Arles (ca. 470–543), saw "fulfilled in the New Testament all the truths which were prefigured in the Old."[25] On the allegorical level, Abraham's sacrifice of Isaac was seen to foreshadow the sacrifice of Jesus by God the Father, the death of Samson was taken as an anticipation of Jesus' passion, and the rod of Moses was understood as the Cross. Joseph's refusal to be seduced by his master's wife was read as the refusal of Christ to submit to the carnal tradition of the synagogue. Abel was interpreted as the chosen Christians and Cain as the rejected Jews—a significance found also in Isaac and Ishmael, Jacob and Esau, Sara and Agar, and Joseph and his brothers. The commentators were often ingenious, inventive, and even extravagant in their search for parallels between the Hebrew and

---

[25] "Sermon 87: On Jacob's Ladder," *Sermons*, trans. Sister Mary Magdeleine Mueller, The Fathers of the Church, XLVII (New York, 1964), 33. For the Latin, see "Sermo LXXXVII: De scala Iacob," *Sermones*, ed. Germanus Morin (Maretioli, 1937), p. 345.

Christian scriptures. Yet if the interpretations appear eso-
teric or excessively imaginative, the method of producing
them was not meant to be beyond the reach of ordinary
men. At the end of one of his explications, Caesarius tells
his audience, "If, with the Lord's help, you will read over
the Sacred Scriptures rather frequently, and heed them
carefully, I believe that you can find an even better explanation."²⁶ And indeed, as Caesarius urged, the allegorical
approach came to be extensively used.

Interpretation through allegorization was widely practiced in the schools, where it was employed to explicate not
only the Old Testament, but also the New Testament and
both pagan and contemporary authors. In addition, the
procedure was used by preachers in homilies and sermons,
so that in time the setting forth of spiritual meanings came
to be a familiar device understood by both educated and
uneducated men. Indeed, as the technique became commonplace, so too did some of its solutions, including the
patristic explanations of the significance of leprosy in the
Bible.

The most frequent early patristic interpretation of leprosy is that it symbolizes heresy.²⁷ Gregory the Great (ca.

²⁶ "Sermon 84: On Abraham and His Son Isaac," *Sermons*, p.
19. For the Latin, see "Sermo LXXXIV: De Abraham et Isaac
filio eius," *Sermones*, p. 333.
²⁷ See Alexander Macalister, "Leprosy," in *A Dictionary of the
Bible*, ed. James Hastings, III (New York, 1901), 98. The connection between leprosy and heresy may have been derived from
the curses in Deuteronomy that are to befall Israel. If it will "not
hear the voice of the Lord thy God, to keep and to do all his
commandments and ceremonies, which I command thee this day,
all these curses shall come upon thee, and overtake thee" (28:15).
Moses states: "Percutiat te Dominus ulcere pessimo in genibus et

540–604), in his *Moralia*, writes that Job's comforters, who delude Job by confusing good and evil, represent heretics who are relieved of their misconceptions through "the preaching and admonition of Holy Church." He finds identical symbolism in the story of the cleansing of the ten lepers (Luke 17:12–19):

For in leprosy both a portion of the skin is brought to a bright hue, and a portion remains of a healthy colour. Lepers therefore are a figure of heretics, for in that they blend evil with good, they cover the complexion of health with spots. And hence that they may be healed, they rightly cry out, *Jesus, Master.*[28]

---

in suris, sanarique non possis a planta pedis usque ad verticem tuum." "May the Lord strike thee with a very sore ulcer in the knees and in the legs, and be thou incurable from the sole of the foot to the top of the head" (28:35). "Very sore ulcer," *ulcus pessimus,* is the term used for Job's disease, whose spread from foot to head is described in the same way as that of the curse: "Egressus igitur Satan a facie Domini percussit Iob ulcere pessimo a planta pedis usque ad verticem eius." "So Satan went forth from the presence of the Lord, and struck Job with a very grievous ulcer, from the sole of the foot even to the top of the head" (Job 2:7). The similarity of phrasing is significant, since early commentators identified Job's disease as leprosy. See *The Interpreter's Bible,* ed. George Arthur Buttrick et al. (New York, 1954), III, 919–920; C. J. Ball, ed. and trans., *The Book of Job* (Oxford, 1922), p. 114.

[28] *Morals on the Book of Job* (I.v.28), A Library of the Fathers of the Holy Catholic Church, XVIII (Oxford, 1844), 262–263. For the Latin, see *Moralium libri,* V.xi.28 (PL, LXXV, 691). The reference here is to a work reprinted in the *Patrologiae cursus completus: Series latina,* ed. J. P. Migne, 221 vols. (Paris, 1844–1880). Citations of writings appearing in Migne first give the title and divisions of the work and second, in parentheses, the volume of the *Patrologia Latina* (PL) and page(s) or column(s) on which the cited portion appears.

Isidore of Seville (ca. 560–636) also interprets the ten lepers as heretics; in the variety of their colors, they exhibit the variety of schisms.[29] Elsewhere, in his commentary on Leviticus 13, Isidore allegorizes leprosy as false doctrine and lepers as heretics, men who profess doctrines of error and confuse true and false. In a minute textual reading accompanied by broad textual interpretation, Isidore identifies the signs of leprosy given in Leviticus with types of heresy. For example, leprosy in flesh and skin (Leviticus 13:3) prefigures the heresy of the Aetians, who insist that they remain in the faith even though they live carnally.[30] The equation between the varieties of leprosy described in Leviticus and particular heretical movements apparently became conventional; Isidore's interpretation is cited, for instance, in the *Glossa Ordinaria*[31] and abstracted in the commentary on the Pentateuch by Bede (ca. 673–735).[32] Finally, one of the most popular medieval handbooks of biblical allegory (incorrectly attributed to Hrabanus Maurus [ca. 780–856] and now assigned to Garner of Rochefort [d. early 13th cent.]) confirms that the association between leprosy and heresy was commonplace. The entry for the words *leprosy* and *lepers* states, "*Leprosy* is sin, or indeed false teaching, as in Leviticus: 'If the stroke of lep-

---

[29] *Allegoriae quaedam Sacrae Scripturae,* 221 (*PL,* LXXXIII, 127).

[30] *Quaestiones in Vetus Testamentum: In Leviticum,* XI (*PL,* LXXXIII, 327–330).

[31] "Liber Leviticus," XIII (*PL,* CXIII, 333). This work is incorrectly attributed by Migne to Walafrid Strabo. The *Glossa Ordinaria* was in fact assembled by various glossators during the twelfth century. See Smalley, pp. 56–66.

[32] "Explanatio in Tertium Librum Mosis," XIII, in *In Pentateuchum Commentarii* (*PL,* XVI, 346–348).

rosy be in a man,' that is, if sin, or heresy, be in a man. *Lepers* are heretics, as in the Gospel [Luke 17:12]: 'There met him ten lepers,' because many come to Christ, who, earlier thinking that the Decalogue had perished, were stained with the filth of heresy."[33]

Of course, the interpreters do not confine the significance of leprosy to a single sin. For instance, although Hrabanus Maurus connects certain types of leprosy with types of heresy, he also links other varieties of leprosy with other sins, such as pride, deceit, hidden blasphemy, anger, hypocrisy, faithlessness, and vices of the flesh.[34] Similarly, a document which sets out to interpret the significance of leprosy as described in Leviticus attaches the various forms of the disease to various sins, including weak faith, fury, rage, the intent to commit homicide, heresy, impure conscience, idolatry, lust, and avarice.[35] Richard of St. Victor (d. 1173), in interpreting Christ's healing of the leper (Matthew 8:1–4), takes the leprosy as a symbol of the many vices which defile mankind spiritually. He states that

fornicators, concubines, the incestuous, adulterers, the avaricious, usurers, false witnesses, perjurers, those likewise who say to a brother, fool, and who look upon a woman concupiscently (who though not evil in deed are nevertheless evil in inclination): all, I say, such as these, who through guilt are cut off from God, all are judged to be leprous by the priests (who know and protect the law of God) and are separated from the company of the faithful, if not physically, nevertheless spiritually.[36]

[33] *Allegoriae in Sacram Scripturam* (PL, CXII, 985).

[34] *De universo*, XVIII.v (PL, CXI, 502).

[35] Saint Jerome, *Scripta supposititia: Epistolae*, XXXIV (PL, XXX, 253–256).

[36] *Allegoriae in Novum Testamentum*, II.xvi (PL, CLXXV, 790).

Moreover, he understands the ten lepers healed by God as "those who live against the precepts of the Ten Commandments, and by different and damnable sins, and by doing evil, they defile themselves."[37]

Among the damnable sins which ecclesiastical writers connect with leprosy, simony and avarice are encountered frequently, particularly in interpretations of the leprosy which strikes Gehazi, the servant of Elisha, who is punished for extracting money and clothing from Naaman (II Kings 5:20–27). Caesarius of Arles finds that Gehazi prefigures Judas: they are alike in that they served their masters avariciously. "Thus we understand that all greedy, avaricious men are covered within their soul with the leprosy of sin."[38] Alain de Lille (1114–1203) states that the leprosy of Naaman which cleaves to Gehazi signifies simony,[39] pre-

---

Though attributed in Migne to Hugh of St. Victor (ca. 1097–1140), this work is now thought to be by Richard of St. Victor.

[37] *Allegoriae in Novum Testamentum*, IV.xxv (*PL*, CLXXV, 823).

[38] "Sermon 129: On Blessed Eliseus and His Servant Giezi," *Sermons*, pp. 228–229. For the Latin, see "Sermo CXXIX: De beato Heliseo et Giezi puero eius," *Sermones*, p. 509.

[39] "Lepra," in *Liber in distinctionibus dictionum theologicalium* (*PL*, CCX, 835). Gehazi's leprosy is alluded to by Gauthier de Châtillon (ca. 1135–after 1189) in the poem "Licet eger cum egrotis":

> Donum Dei non donatur,
> nisi gratis conferatur;
> quod qui vendit vel mercatur,
> lepra Syri vulneratur.   [25–28]

(The gift of God is not given unless given for nothing; he who sells and buys is maimed with Syrian leprosy.)

See *Die Gedichte Walters von Chatillon*, ed. Karl Strecker (Berlin, 1925), p. 46.

sumably because both Gehazi and Simon Magus (Acts 8:14–24) viewed sacred things as suitable for purchase and sale.⁴⁰

It is not surprising that the commentators also link leprosy with sexual depravity. Lust was one of the deadly sins, and what is more, leprosy was commonly assumed to be a venereal disease.⁴¹ In accordance with that notion, Adamus Scotus (fl. 1180) writes that Naaman the leper falls to pride and from pride into lust, "for what is the impurity of leprosy, unless it is the sin of lust?"⁴² Tertullian (ca. 160–after 220) interprets leprosy as a metaphor for adultery in his argument that the apostles did not promise a second penitence to the unchaste. Just as the biblical law (in Leviticus 13:14) states that when old leprous flesh appears, the patient must be pronounced defiled, "so also is adultery an irremovable blemish when it returns once more from the past and sullies the purity of that new coloring from which it was effaced."⁴³ Prudentius (348–after 405), in his *Peristephanon*,⁴⁴ attaches leprosy to carnal sin in his

⁴⁰ Richard of St. Victor, *Allegoriae in Vetus Testamentum*, VII.xxix (*PL*, CLXXV, 720). The work is incorrectly attributed by Migne to Hugh of St. Victor.

⁴¹ See Chapter I.

⁴² *Sermones*, XLV (*PL*, CXCVIII, 411).

⁴³ *On Purity*, 20 in *Treatises on Penance: On Penitence and On Purity*, trans. William P. Le Saint, Ancient Christian Writers, no. 28 (Westminster, Maryland, 1959), pp. 116–117. For the Latin, see *De pudicitia*, XX (*PL* II, 1075–76).

⁴⁴ *Prudentius*, ed. and trans. H. J. Thomson, The Loeb Classical Library, II (Cambridge, Mass., 1953), 98–345. Further references to this poem, which are all line numbers of the poem's second book, are given in parentheses or brackets. Translations are from the pages facing the Latin.

description of one who is morally deformed by spiritual leprosy:

> istum libido foetida
> per scorta tractum publica
> luto et cloacis inquinat,
> dum spurca mendicat stupra.   [245–248]

> (This other is dragged by foul lust among public harlots and polluted with mire and filth as he goes a-begging after dirty whorings.)

This description comes in a passage that characterizes self-seeking, worldly men as leprous in their souls. Though physically healthy, they have "sores on soul and character," and their "blood is hot for sin" (223–224, 213):

> vestros valentes corpore
> interna corrumpit lepra,
> errorque mancum claudicat
> et caeca fraus nihil videt.   [229–232]

> (But yours [i.e., proud, worldly men] while strong in body, are corrupted by an inner leprosy, their superstition halts like one that is maimed, their self-deception is blind and sightless.)

The leprous sinners described by Prudentius are not all sexually depraved. What is common to all, however, is their profane worldliness and the leprosy that symbolizes it.[45]

---

[45] Prudentius' characterizations of those "corrupted by an inner leprosy" seem to describe men suffering from diseases distinct from leprosy. For instance, the prideful man has "a watery dropsy of the soul within"—*hydrops aquosus* (239), or edema. The rulers of Rome suffer from "the ruler's sickness"—*morbus regis* (264),

Appropriately, the avaricious man has hands that permanently grasp:[46]

> ast hic avarus contrahit
> manus recurvas et volam
> plicans aduncis unguibus
> laxare nervos non valet.   [241–244]

> (And here is another who in his greed crooks his hands and draws them close, his palm doubled, his fingernails like hooks, and cannot relax the tendons.)

One sinner, who hotly seeks for advancement in rank, pants with fevers and is "maddened by the fire in his veins" (249–252). Another, who cannot keep a secret, "suffers tortures from the irritation of his passion and the constant itch in his heart" (253–256). The envious have "scrofulous swellings," and the angry show the "discoloured festering sores of malice" (257–260). The leprous symptoms of Prudentius' sinners—the sexuality, edema, jaundice, maiming, blindness, claw hands, itching, fevers, swelling, and ulcerations—externalize the spiritual effects of their sinfulness. The passage that ends the description of them emphasizes the hideousness of their depravity:

---

or jaundice. Edema and jaundice were recognized by Celsus as diseases separate from leprosy, but both conditions were understood by medieval physicians to accompany leprosy. Theodoric of Cervia states that a sign of alopecian leprosy is edema and that leonine leprosy produces "yellowishness of the face," a principle sign of jaundice. Moreover, each of the sinners described by Prudentius is one of "your great men" (233), one of "yours . . . corrupted by an inner leprosy" (229–230). In short, all those described in II.221–228 are deformed in different ways by leprosy.

46 The description seems to be of the complication of leprosy known as the claw hand malformation. See Chapter I.

peccante nil est taetrius,
nil tam leprosum aut putidum;
cruda est cicatrix criminum
oletque ut antrum Tartari.   [285–288]

(There is nothing fouler than a sinner, nothing so leprous or rotten; the wound of his sins keeps bleeding and
stinks like the pit of hell.)

Thus, for Prudentius, leprosy is finally not merely tied to
sexual excess, or avariciousness, or anger. It is the symbol
of sinfulness, of general ethical decay.

Leprosy is commonly used as a figure of generalized sin.
In explaining the significance of Leviticus 14:49–53, Justin
Martyr (ca. 103–ca. 165) writes that the leprosy is to be
understood as "an emblem of sin."[47] Rupert of Deutz (ca.
1070–1129 [1135?]) interprets Naaman's bathing in the
Jordan as a prefiguration of the cleansing of sin through
baptism.[48] Isidore of Seville writes that the leper cured by
Christ (Matthew 8:1–4) represents "the human race defiled
with the contagion of sin."[49] Tertullian, commenting on
Luke 5:12–14, explains that the leper is "a person who was
defiled with sins."[50] And in one of the most important

[47] *The Writings of Justin Martyr and Athenagoras*, trans. Marcus Dods, George Reith, and B. P. Pratten, The Ante-Nicene
Christian Library, II (Edinburgh, 1870), 357.

[48] *De trinitate et operibus ejus: In Libros Regum liber quintus*,
XXIX (*PL*, CLXVII, 1263). See also Caesarius, *Sermons*, pp. 229–
230 (*Sermones*, p. 510). Interestingly, the common equation of
leprosy and sin is reflected in certain medieval legends that describe
the healing of leprosy through baptism. See Alfred Maury, *Croyances et légendes du Moyen Age* (Paris, 1896), p. 153.

[49] *Allegoriae quaedam Sacrae Scripturae*, 150 (*PL*, LXXXIII,
118).

[50] *The Five Books of Quintus Sept. Flor. Tertullianus Against*

medieval commentaries on Leviticus, Radulphus Flaviacensis (middle of twelfth century) offers an interpretation
of the spiritual significance of leprosy which crystallizes
the medieval view of the disease. In the opening paragraphs
of his commentary on Leviticus 13 and 14, he identifies
lepers as those who, in keeping with the devil's perversity,
sin and intend to sin without regret for their sins. "For
those are men whom the law describes as lepers and whom
it decrees be separated from the camp of the holy. Provision must be made so that the sick do not infect the healthy
through frequent familiarity and daily conversations, for the
sick refuse to put aside their disease through stubborn tenac-
ity. And so the law names as lepers not those who have
sinned, but those who have sinned and not repented." In the
commentary which follows, Radulphus sets out the corre-
spondences between the various types of leprosy described
in Leviticus and particular kinds of sin. Leprosy of the
head and beard signifies corrupt faith; leprous ulcers in the
flesh and skin are caused by crimes and vices, such as the
intemperance associated with the adulteries of David (II
Kings 11) and Herod (Mark 6:17–18); and leprosy in a
woolen or linen garment is the leprosy of one "consumed
by depravity of virtue, which is either the allurement of
flesh or infidelity."[51] For Radulphus, all the forms of biblical leprosy are variations on a single moral failure: the
denial of the Church and its laws. He writes, "Whoever

Marcion, trans. Peter Holmes, The Ante-Nicene Christian Library,
III (Edinburgh, 1870), 200. For the Latin, see *Adversus Marcionem
Libri Quinque*, IV.ix (*PL* II, 403).

[51] Radulphus Flaviacensis, *Commentatiorum in Leuiticum Libri
XX*, ed. Margarino de la Bigne, Maxima Bibliotheca Vetervm
Patrvm, et Antiqvorvm Scriptorvm Ecclesiasticorvm (London,
1677), XVII, 130, 134, 139.

has been corrupted by the disease of spiritual leprosy, as either by the offense of faithlessness or because of depravity of morals, should be sequestered from association with the faithful, for it is established that such a one does not hold to the laws of the Church, and through this separation having been imposed, he will be anything to himself, easily moving others to scorn him."[52]

The view of leprosy taken by Radulphus and the other Christian biblical commentators cited here is duplicated elsewhere in the writings of the commentators, for the medieval interpreters of leprosy differ from each other primarily in detail rather than conception. They variously connect scriptural leprosy with heresy, cupidity, pride, absence or weakness of faith, carnal sin, the sins of the Decalogue, the cardinal sins, and with sin itself; but they all accept the premise enunciated by Radulphus. Citations from the commentaries could be greatly extended beyond what has been presented here, but an accumulation of passages on leprosy would hardly alter—and would indeed emphasize—the central observation to be made about the exegetes' handling of leprosy: they are all agreed that leprosy signifies denial of divine law.

The influence of this exegetical premise on the popular conception of leprosy as a disease with moral connotations was surely substantial. Consider that an observation made by Prudentius in his *Peristephanon* is echoed nine centuries later by Saint Louis (1215–1270). Prudentius asks,

> carnisne morbus foedior,
> an mentis et morum ulcera?   [223–224]

---

[52] Radulphus, p. 138.

(Is disease of the flesh more loathsome, or the sores on soul and character?)

and concludes that "there is nothing fouler than a sinner, nothing so leprous or rotten." Compare a conversation between Louis and Jean de Joinville. Louis asks Jean if he would prefer to be a leper or to commit a mortal sin. When Jean admits that he would rather commit thirty sins than be a leper, Louis rebukes him: "For you ought to know that there is no leprosy as ugly as the leprosy of being in mortal sin, because the soul that is in mortal sin is like the devil."[53]

The idea of moral leprosy first elaborated by the Church fathers is seen again and again in medieval writing, such as preacher's handbooks and homilies. It is found in the *Manuel des Péchés:*

> Chescun en peché mortel
> Est vn leprus espirituel.   [9891–9892]

(Each one in deadly sin is a spiritual leper.)

and in an English translation of that work:

> He þat ys yn dedly synne,
> Gostely he ys a mesyl with-ynne.   [11465–11466][54]

[53] Jean, Sire de Joinville, *Histoire de Saint Louis,* IV.27 in *Histoire de Saint Louis, Credo, et Lettre à Louis X,* ed. and trans. Natalis de Wailly, 2d ed. (Paris, 1874), pp. 14–15. Cf. the similar remark in the *Ancrene Wisse:* "May God know this—and he does know it—I would prefer you all to have leprosy than to have you envious or with hatred in your hearts." See *Ancrene Wisse: The English Text of the Ancrene Riwle,* ed. J. R. R. Tolkien, EETS, no. 249 (London, 1962), p. 128.

[54] Robert Mannyng of Brunne, *Robert of Brunne's "Handlyng Synne," A.D. 1303, with Those Parts of the Anglo-French Treatise*

It also appears in the preacher's manual by Pierre Bersuire
(ca. 1290–1362), who observes that just as four kinds of
physical leprosy are matched with the four humors,[55] so
spiritual leprosy is associated with four sins: simony, pride,
avarice, and sexual impurity.[56] Furthermore, the joining of
leprosy and mortal sin is conventional in sermons, such as
those on Matthew 8:1–4. A thirteenth-century German
sermon identifies the leper healed by Christ as the type of
man who is defiled by deadly sins,[57] and a French homily
(ca. 1170) by Maurice of Sully lists the sorts of sins sym-
bolized by the leprosy:

The leper signifies sinners, and the leprosy the sins . . . the
great damnable sins, such as fornication, adultery, usury,
robbery, theft, gluttony, drunkenness, and all those sins by
which a man is damned and sure to lose the love of God and
his friends. . . . Through leprosy a man is cut off from the
company of people, and through deadly sins a man is cut off
from the company of God and Holy Church, for he who dies

---

on which It was Founded, William of Wadington's "Manuel des
Pechiez," ed. Frederick J. Furnivall, EETS, O.S., nos. 119, 123
(London, 1901, 1903), p. 357.

[55] For an instance of such matching in a medieval medical
writer, see Theodoric's use of humoral theory, Chapter I. Cf. "Leviticus," *Midrash Rabbah*, IV, 190: "Man is evenly balanced, half
of him is water, and the other half is blood. When he is deserving
the water does not exceed the blood, nor does the blood exceed
the water; but when he sins, it sometimes happens that the water
gains over the blood and he then becomes a sufferer from dropsy;
at other times the blood gains over the water and he then becomes leprous."

[56] *Repertorium, vulgo Dictionarium morale*, in *Opera omnia
totam S. Scripturae* . . . (Antwerp, 1609), III, 909–910.

[57] *Altdeutsche Predigten*, ed. Anton E. Schönbach, III (Graz,
1891), 37.

in deadly sin is cut off from the company of God and his angels.[58]

The French homilist approaches his text as other writers of sermons frequently do. Typically, the biblical portion is given in Latin and then retold in the vernacular. The interpretation of the passage begins with the typing of the leper as sinner, his leprosy as sins. Next the preacher names specific sins represented by the leprosy. In this way, a northern English metrical homily on Matthew 8:1–4 opens its interpretation by explaining that the physical disease is a sign of moral impurity, and proceeds to make the immorality specific:

> And herbi wille the maister mene,
> That mankind hafd noht ben mad clen
> Of sin, bot Crist haued comen doun
> Fra heuen, to gif for man ranzoun.

[58] *Maurice of Sully and the Medieval Vernacular Homily: With the Text of Maurice's French Homilies from a Sens Cathedral Chapter MS.*, ed. C. A. Robson (Oxford, 1952), p. 91. The same list of sins is attached to a sermon on Luke 17:11–19 (the healing of the ten lepers), though the list there also includes "perjury, fraud, homicide, calling one's neighbor a fool or dolt, or looking at a woman with the intention of coveting her for evil work" (p. 155). The passage is obviously analogous to one by Richard of St. Victor, quoted earlier in this chapter. Richard's mention of those "qui etiam dicunt fratri, fatue, et qui vidunt mulierem ad concupiscendam eam," is clearly matched in Maurice's "clamer son proisme fol u musart u esgarder fame por li covoitier por malvaise uevre." (The French reading of Latin *frater* as "neighbor" [*proisme*] rather than as "brother" accurately translates one of the Latin meanings.) Robson (p. 198, note to homily 4) cites other similar texts in Hugh and Richard of St. Victor. For a thirteenth-century English translation of Maurice's sermon on Luke, see *An Old English Miscellany*, ed. Richard Morris, EETS, O.S., no. 49 (London, 1872), p. 31.

For man quaim sinne mad unhale,
Haft noht ben bette of his bale,
Bot yef Crist haued til him comen,
And his seknes opon him nomen,
And clensed him of leper of sinne,
That alle mankind was fallen in.
For riht als leper mas bodi
Ugli, and lathe, and unherly,
Sua mas the filth of licheri,
The sawel ful lath, gastelye,
And the bolning of priue pride
Es leper, that na man mai hide.
And eft and nythe and felounye
Mai be cald leper gastilie,
And couaitis of symounye,
That was wel sen on Gyseye.[59]

(And by this the master [i.e., Matthew] intends that mankind would not have been made clean of sin unless Christ had come down from heaven to give ransom for man. For man, whom sin made unhealthy, would not have been assuaged of his misfortune unless Christ had come to him, and taken his sickness upon Himself, and cleansed him of the leprosy of sin, that all mankind had fallen into. For just as leprosy makes the body ugly, loathsome, and monstrous, so the filth of lechery makes the soul very loathsome spiritually, and the swelling of secret pride is leprosy, that no man may hide. And envy and malice and wickedness may be called spiritual leprosy, and covetousness of simony, that was well seen in Gehazi.)

[59] *English Metrical Homilies: From Manuscripts of the Fourteenth Century*, ed. John Small (Edinburgh, 1862), pp. 129–130.

It is not difficult to see that Maurice of Sully and the author of the English homily are bearers of the same message. They may illustrate moral leprosy with different transgressions, yet their homilies contain significant resemblances, not only in form but also in content. The preachers emphasize that the leprosy represents sins which damn, and the sins they name can be located in the commentaries which underlie their sermons. True, it is not always possible to trace a homily back to one source, but nevertheless the transgressions the homily associates with leprosy can usually be found distributed among several patristic writers. The sermon by Maurice of Sully, which apparently derives from Richard of St. Victor, is certainly not an isolated example of a sermon with patristic origins. When Saint Anthony of Padua (1195–1231) types the ten lepers as the human race marked by its violation of the Ten Commandments, he is repeating an idea found in the fathers; and when he goes on to equate ten types of leprosy named in Leviticus with ten types of sin (hypocrisy, ambition for transitory dignities, impurity of lust, graft and usury, envy, impurity of thought, open iniquity, disorder of life, abandonment of the Christian faith, and discord),[60] he is working a variation on a patristic theme. It has been said of Anthony's sermons that they are a "font and treasure of [his] theological, patristical, and biblical knowledge." He quotes Augustine, Bernard, Gregory the Great, Jerome, Isidore, Ambrose, Origen, Bede, John Damascene, Hrabanus Maurus, and—with particular frequency—the glossaries which compile the in-

[60] "Dominica XIV. post Trinitatem," *Sermones*, pp. 276–277 in *Sancti Francisci Assisiatis . . . nec non S. Antonii Paduani . . . Opera omnia . . .*, ed. Joannes de la Haye (Stadt am Hof, 1739).

terpretations of these and other writers.[61] Accordingly, like Maurice's, Anthony's sermons communicated the ideas of the patristic exegetes to the unlearned.[62] Indeed, the medieval homilists in general were the disseminators of the patristic understandings of leprosy: through preachers' manuals, sermon collections, and devotional writings, they conveyed to the popular culture the ecclesiastical idea of moral leprosy.

The *Gesta Romanorum*, an anthology of entertaining stories intended for inclusion in sermons, indicates how thoroughly the commonplaces of patristic exegesis merged with popular culture. The stories of the *Gesta Romanorum* were meant to help a preacher engage the attention of an audience of common people. The tales therefore often appeal to the taste for the improbable, bizarre, scandalous, or fabulous; in them, one encounters dragons, adulteresses, evil seneschals, talking animals, demons, and much else. Of course, these stories—interesting as they are in themselves —all contain hidden moral significances, which the preacher explains by ingenious, or at least extravagant, allegorization. For example, there is a tale involving a noble knight named Iosias. One day while he is asleep, Iosias' wife steps outside and forgets to lock the door. A bear enters and bathes in the well, causing the water to be infected with venom. Iosias, his wife, and all their men drink the water

[61] Raphael M. Huber, *St. Anthony of Padua, Doctor of the Church Universal* (Milwaukee, 1948), pp. 76–78.

[62] It is true that Anthony's are in Latin, but as often happened with collections of Latin sermons, they became a source for preachers who translated them into the vernacular. See *St. Anthony of Padua*, p. 76, and G. R. Owst, *Preaching in Medieval England: An Introduction to Sermon Manuscipts of the Period c. 1350–1450* (Cambridge, Eng., 1926), pp. 223 ff.

and are poisoned with "synfull lepr." What does this signify? The flesh of even a good Christian man leaves the door open to the devil, who puts the venom of sin into the well of mercy, causing the flesh and all that is sinful to be infected.[63] In another story, a king puts his only daughter into the care of a guardian, and warns the man to keep her from drinking from a particular fountain whose water causes leprosy. However, the daughter does drink from it and naturally becomes leprous. The cure is revealed by a hermit, who directs the girl to hit a certain stone with a rod, so that moisture will come out of the stone. When she applies the moisture to herself, she is cured. The lesson: the world (the fountain) infects the soul (the daughter) with sin (leprosy), but the Church (the hermit) shows that sin can be removed through penitence (the rod) and the tears of a contrite heart (the moisture).[64]

Whether those two stories were written as moral allegories or whether allegorizations were appended to existing stories, the writer was using a symbol which lay ready at hand. Wherever leprosy appears in the *Gesta Romanorum*, it is connected with sin—and indeed is usually a figure for sin itself.

When a preacher's congregation gathered to hear him condemn sin, they might hear the story of the leper healed by Christ or of the one cured by swallowing a serpent in a cup of wine[65] interpreted as a parable of Christ's grace in

[63] "LXII. Solemius a Wyse Emperore," *The Early English Version of the Gesta Romanorum*, ed. Sidney J. H. Herrtage, EETS, E.S., no. 33 (London, 1879), pp. 263–268.

[64] Tale XCIV, *Gesta Romanorum: Entertaining Moral Stories*, trans. Charles Swan (London, 1905), pp. 218–219.

[65] Tale CLI, *Gesta Romanorum*, trans. Swan, p. 297.

forgiving repentant sinners. On another day, the preacher might allegorize an Old Testament story—about Gehazi or Miriam, for example—and use the leprosy as a figure for simony or some other sin, of for the deadly sins. And the more sermons they would hear, the more completely would the congregation receive the moral associations of leprosy as elaborated by ecclesiastical writers and transmitted by the preacher.

If the influence of the homiletic tradition upon the popular attitude toward leprosy was significant, its influence upon the attitude of medieval poets was no less so, for poets, like other men, were affected by preachers—just as they were by doctors' diagnoses, mayors' edicts, civil and ecclesiastical law, and stories told in taverns. It is therefore to be expected that their use of leprosy would reflect the popular conceptions of the disease. Each time a poet uses leprosy as a physical symbol of an inner moral condition, he expects that his audience will understand the moral significance of the disease. The figure in a story who becomes leprous because he perjures himself, or because he glories in worldly success, or because he is lustful—all these are moral examples in a popular moral tradition.

The poets undoubtedly took the idea of leprosy as a punishment for fraud primarily, perhaps exclusively, from the ecclesiastical tradition. Richard of St. Victor and Maurice of Sully speak of false witnesses and perjurers as spiritual lepers, Hrabanus Maurus connects leprosy with deceit, and the physician Guy of Chauliac characterizes lepers as "schemers and deceivers." Likewise, pride is among the sins connected with leprosy by Hrabanus, Pierre Bersuire, the author of the English metrical homily, and the homilists who remind sinners that Azariah was struck with leprosy in punishment for his presumption.[66] Similarly, Moses' leprosy could be taken to demonstrate that pride in one's actions is as loathsome to God as leprosy is loathsome to men.[67]

While the poets received the connection of leprosy and pride solely from ecclesiastical writers, it is an oversimplification to suggest that the same sort of influence affected their use of the link between leprosy and lust. Leprosy is frequently interpreted by them as carnal sin—so frequently, in fact, that Pierre Bersuire observes that, while leprosy can signify any sin, it especially represents the sin of lust.[68] But this emphasis can be traced to the same influence that works on the poets—a pervasive cultural understanding. The Jewish exegetes state that leprosy can be a punishment for gross unchastity, public edicts warn that lepers frequent houses of prostitution, and medical writers observe both that the disease can be venereal in origin and that it excites sexual desire. Thus, the connection between leprosy and carnality is ubiquitous in medieval culture, and the religious, medical, and popular understandings of leprosy influence and reinforce each other. Consequently, a homiletic writer could be expected to reproduce the common assertion that the leper is a person with coarse sexual needs. It is this depravity, presumably, which lies behind one of the

[66] For example, see *Middle English Sermons*, ed. Woodburn O. Ross, EETS, O.S., no. 209 (London, 1940), p. 211. The poet Lydgate refers to this instance also. See *Lydgate's Fall of Princes*, book V, ll. 2299–2312, ed. Henry Bergen, Carnegie Institute of Washington, no. 262 (Washington, 1923), II, 649.

[67] *Ancrene Wisse*, pp. 77 f.

[68] *Reductorium morale, super totam Bibliam*, III.6 *in Opera omnia*, II, 47.

three reasons Robert Mannyng offers for not having sexual intercourse with common women:

> Þe þredde ys þe werste wem;
> Meseles, men seye, vsen hem;
> And, who takeþ hem yn þat hete,
> Clennesse of body he may sone lete.[69]

(The third is the worst blemish: men say lepers use them, and he who takes them in that heat may soon forsake purity of body.)

The influence of the popular connection between leprosy and wanton sexuality is seen in a number of ways in sermons. Even though the disease might not be explicitly connected with lust, it could nevertheless be understood as if it had been. The *Gesta Romanorum* contains a story about a woman who contracts leprosy from a knight and then infects a prince with the disease.[70] The moralization reveals that the story is about how the soul is infected with sin by the devil, and how Christ takes upon Himself the sinful nature of mankind. "The leprosy is iniquity," the preacher explains. He doesn't need to explain that it is also a venereal disease. In the tale, the knight wilfully infects the woman with the leprosy, for she is more beautiful than his own wife, who is deformed and hateful. In order to "remove the disparity" between the two women, "the envious knight instantly infected himself with leprosy, and communicated the disease to the lady." The lady is told that the remedy for her illness is to stand in the main thoroughfare of a large city and play the role of a

[69] *Handlyng Synne*, ll. 7447–7450.
[70] Tale CLI, *Gesta Romanorum*, trans. Swan, pp. 296–297.

whore; the disease will be transferred to whoever takes her first.[71] It is obvious that the story assumes the medical belief in the leper as the bearer of a venereal disease which is easily spread through promiscuous sexual intercourse.

Another tale in the *Gesta Romanorum* similarly links leprosy with carnal sin. In the story of Merelaus the emperor, Merelaus decides to visit the Holy Land; he places his wife in control of his land, with his brother as steward under her. In the emperor's absence, the brother tries to seduce the empress, who steadfastly refuses him. She finally must have her brother-in-law thrown in prison, but after a time he appears to repent and is released. Shortly afterward, the empress and her steward ride out in the forest with a group of retainers, but they are separated from the company. The steward sees his chance: "And when he saw that, he said, 'Dame, here next to us is a private forest, and I have loved you for a long time; let us go there now, and let me play with you.'" She rejects him again, and in his passion he strips her bare of all her clothing save her smock, and hangs her by the hair on an oak. She survives and is rescued, and after various encounters with other men who threaten her, she enters a nunnery. Meanwhile, "the brother of her husband, who hung her by the hair, was a foul leper," and the others who mistreated her are also, though differently, afflicted. The interpretation explains that the story is an allegory of the soul placed in danger by the wretched flesh (the brother), which strips a soul of its good

[71] In Swan's translation, the idea that the leprosy can be transferred is only suggested; the point is made explicit in a Latin version other than Swan's. See *Die Gesta Romanorum*, ed. Wilhelm Dick, *Erlanger Beiträge zur Englischen Philologie*, VII (1890), 206. Presumably, the idea is a folk belief.

virtues and hangs it on worldly love. But the soul turns from wordly vanities to holy life, and so the threat to the soul is overcome. At no point is the leprosy said to be connected with sin, although the character of the emperor's brother makes it very clear that his leprosy is a punishment for his actions. The brother is stricken not with just any disease, but with the appropriate disease, the one that suits his crime, and so are the other tormentors of the empress.[72] Leprosy afflicts the brother because he is a lustful man, and it is fitting that he should be struck with the disease of such a sinner. There is poetic justice here, and the medieval audience knew it.

In sum, the medieval poets inherited an ancient and pervasive tradition that branded the leper as a pariah. It accused him of being immoral, separated him from society, took him as a figure of sin, feared him for the disease he spread and for the terror he inspired. It is this background that shapes the literary representation of the leper as a man who is morally depraved, whose body bears the stain of his spiritual corruption.

[72] "Merelaus þe Emperour," *The Early English Versions of the Gesta Romanorum*, pp. 313–322.

IV

Leprosy in Literature

"My leprosie is a defiled soule."
Samuel Rowlands,
The Betraying of Christ

Society recognized in the leper's physical corruption the mark of moral corruption. For the physician, the mere presence of the disease might well bespeak the possibility of sinful acts. A priest, out of charity, and remembering the verse in Isaiah which told of Jesus' leprosy, might not be as ready as the doctor to say that one of his neighbors must have sinned. Yet at the ceremony which separated the leper from the world, he would tell the poor man that God wished to punish him for the evil he had done in this world. Likewise, in a sermon, he would explain that Jesus coming down from the mountain to heal the leper was the savior coming from heaven to redeem sinful man. There were few in the parish who did not attach the immorality of the leper in the Bible to the lepers outside the town gate. Why shouldn't they, after all? The king had warned that for their own solace the lepers were spreading the disease among the healthy, and everyone knew that the lepers were driven by a depraved and irresistable sexual urge. The disease was emblematic of a vice-ridden soul.

The writer who introduced a leper into his work surely understood that leprosy was not simply an illness. It was a punishment sent by God, as the poets Bodel and Fastoul knew when they were struck by leprosy. The illness was the dreadful manifestation of an inner disease, a disease of the soul. A writer would naturally use leprosy as a symbol of moral guilt, as Hartmann von Aue does in *Der Arme Heinrich* (ca. 1195), for example.

Hartmann introduces Heinrich as a man apparently beyond blame. He possesses all the virtues a knight should have:

> an dem enwas vergezzen
> nie deheiner der tugent
> die ein ritter in sîner jugent
> ze vollem lobe haben sol.   [32–35]¹

(There was not missing in him any of the chivalric excellence that a knight should have for full praise in his youth.)

He has high birth and wealth, and in addition to those things, honor and knightly spirit, *êre* and *muot* (38–46). He obtains the praise of other men; his reputation is unparalleled:

> man sprach dô nieman alsô wol
> in allen den landen.
>
> . . . . .
>
> alsus kund er gewinnen
> der werlte lop unde pris.   [36–37, 72–73]

(No one then in all the world was spoken of so well.

---

¹ All quotations are taken from Hartman von Aue, *Der Arme Heinrich*, ed. Erich Gierach and J. Knight Bostock, 4th ed. (Oxford, 1965). Line references are given in parentheses or brackets.

. . . Thus he was able to obtain the praise of worldly society and esteem.)

As Hartmann takes pains to emphasize (his opening description of Heinrich's pefection runs to more than forty lines), his hero presents the appearance of unflawed virtue to the world. And truly he is a perfect knight in all things —in all things, that is, but one: he does not serve, or even acknowledge, God.

Heinrich is a man separated by his worldly concerns from God. The adjective consistently used to describe him is *werltlich,* worldly:

> im was der rehte wunsch gegeben
> von werltlîchen êren.   [56–57]

(The complete perfection of worldly honor was given to him.)

The praise he wins is *werlte lop* (73), worldly praise, and he savors *werltlîcher wünne* (79), worldly joy. It is said of him:

> er was ein bluome der jugent,
> der werltfroüde ein spiegelglas.   [60–61]

(He was the bloom of youth, a mirror of worldly joy.)

Werlt, of course, is this world, not the other, more durable one, and Heinrich does not see that he places faith in perishable things, in a world whose very essence is transience:

> Dirre werlte veste,
> ir staete und ir beste
> und ir groeste magenkraft,
> diu stât âne meisterschaft.   [97–100]

(The strength of this world, its constancy and its best
and greatest might, stand deprived of control.)

He does not see that he sins through his concern for reputation in this world and his disregard of the next. He does
not know he is corrupted by vainglory,[2] and for his pride,
his *hôchmuot* (82), his *übermuot* (404), God afflicts him
with leprosy.[3]

Heinrich is punished because of his total absorption in
the secular and his disregard of the sacred. God casts him
down from his state of secular perfection, just as He did
Absalom (II Samuel 13–19), who was also taught not to
trust in *werltlîcher süeze*, worldly sweetness (82–90).[4] Like
Absalom, Heinrich must be made to recognize his guilt,
and leprosy is perfectly suited to chastize him. The disease
destroys all that he has achieved, all that is most important
to him—his worldly honor. At God's command, he falls
into disgrace, *in ein smaelîchez leit* (118); he grows re-
pugnant to all men—he who formerly was attractive to the

[2] According to Chaucer's Parson, who terms it a twig of pride,
"Veyneglorie is for to have pompe and delit in his temporeel
hynesse, and glorifie hym in this worldly estaat" (ParsT, 405, in
The Works of Geoffrey Chaucer, ed. F. N. Robinson, 2d ed. [Bos-
ton, 1957]).

[3] Hartmann's depiction of Heinrich leaves no doubt that Heinrich is chastized for his pride, as comments on the poem demonstrate. See Werner Fechter, "Uber den 'Armen Heinrich' Hartmanns von Aue," *Euphorion*, XLIX (1955), 3–4; Bert Nagel, *Der
Arme Heinrich Hartmanns von Aue: Eine Interpretation* (Tübingen, 1952), pp. 45–46; H. B. Willson, "Symbol and Reality in
'Der Arme Heinrich,'" *MLR*, LIII (1958), 527. The poem reflects
the traditional tie between leprosy and pride in ecclesiastical and
homiletic writing.

[4] Church literature cites Absalom as an example of sinful ambition. That Heinrich does not have the correct attitude toward
God is emphasized by the Absalom parallel. See Fechter, pp. 3 f.

world becomes unpleasant to see or even hear of (124–127).
The first stage of Heinrich's punishment is thereby accomplished:

> sîn hôchmuot wart verkêret
> in ein leben gar geneiget.   [82–83]

(His pride was changed into a completely humbled life.)

But his spiritual rebirth is still to come. He must recognize
his guilt, submit himself to God, and thus finally be
cleansed of leprosy, the symbol of his secular arrogance.

That Heinrich does not immediately recognize God's
supremacy over temporal things is shown by his efforts to
discover a cure by consulting physicians. He travels to
Montpellier, only to learn he cannot be healed. From there
he goes to Salerno, where a physician tells him that, although there is a cure, it is unobtainable: Heinrich will
remain unhealed unless God Himself becomes the physician
(203–204). But Heinrich refuses to bend his will to God's.
If he can himself obtain a remedy, he will, and so he demands that the physician reveal to him what must be done.
When Heinrich learns that the medical cure depends upon
a young girl's sacrificing herself for him, he concludes
that indeed he must remain a leper. Hence, by disregarding
the possibility of a healing through divine grace, Heinrich
accentuates his separation from God.

In despair of a cure, Heinrich distributes his property
among friends, needy strangers, and religious houses,

> daz sich got erbarmen
> geruochte über der sêle heil.   [254–255]

(that God might be pleased to take pity on the health
of his soul.)

The charity Heinrich shows is admirable, but it is flawed, for just as he tried to buy his physical cure from the physician at Salerno with gold and silver (208–213), he now tries to purchase the salvation of his soul. He fails to understand that some things cannot be bought but must be earned.

Having disposed of his wealth, Heinrich retires to a woodland farm which he leases to a peasant. After three years pass, the farmer asks him whether any cure is possible, and Heinrich explains the significance of his disease. God has punished him, he says, because he indulged himself in *werltlicher wünne* (387) and was a *werlttôre*, a fool who believed he could possess honor and wealth without acknowledging God (395–399). Thus, through his disease, he has reached a moral awareness of his sinfulness, but he has not yet accepted the full import of his leprosy. God has punished him, he continues, and the cure can be obtained only if a virgin will spill her blood for him,[5]

[5] The tradition of healing leprosy by blood, particularly the blood of children, is seen in early Hebrew biblical commentary, Pliny, and many texts of the Middle Ages. In Hartmann, as elsewhere, the moral significance of the cure is apparent. Typically, in clinical practice, the medieval doctor would attempt to treat a condition with remedies containing qualities inimical to the sickness. For example, a man with excess hot and moist humors would be given a cold and dry remedy. Likewise, Heinrich's disease, which stems from moral impurity, can be cured by an antidote of high purity—the blood of a virgin. Elsewhere, as in the Amis and Amiloun story, the blood of innocent children is named as a cure. Thus, for writers who understand leprosy to be a moral disease, the cure by blood can be effective only if the donor is morally pure. The blood cure plays a part in literature because it is symbolically significant, not because the poets sought to depict actual medical practices. The motif has been widely studied, and the bibliography on the subject is large. See *Amis and Amiloun*, ed. MacEdward Leach, EETS, O.S., no. 203 (London, 1937),

und mir waer niht anders guot
wan von ir herzen daz bluot.   [450–451]

(and nothing else would be good for me except the
blood from her heart.)

He still refuses to admit God's power to save as well as
destroy, still insists that his cure is to be found solely in
this world. He is still a *werlttôre*.

Hartmann emphasizes the enormity of Heinrich's spiritual failure by contrasting it with the innocence of the
peasant's daughter, the child who helps bring about his
purification. The contrast is at once physical and spiritual,
for just as Heinrich is defiled in body and soul, so the
maiden is pure both ways. One has only to compare the
characterization of Heinrich with the child's estimation of
herself as she convinces her parents to let her be sacrificed.
If Heinrich understands things from the point of view of a
werlttôre, if his ambitions are strictly secular, those of the
innocent girl are strictly sacred. Her argument to her
parents is that life is lived at the cost of the soul and she is
as yet still pure (668–692), untouched by *werltlich gelust*
(690), worldly lust; let her sacrifice herself before she sins
so that she may obtain salvation.

ich wil mich alsus reine
antwürten in gotes gewalt.   [698–699]

(Thus pure, I wish to surrender myself to God's power.)

---

p. lxii, n. 1; Paul Remy, "La lèpre, thème littéraire au moyen âge:
Commentaire d'un passage du roman provençal de Jaufré," *MA*,
LII (1946), 210–233; and Paulus Cassel, *Die Symbolik des Blutes
und "Der arme Heinrich" von Hartmann von Aue* (Berlin, 1882).
Bostock, *Der Arme Heinrich*, p. xxix, calls attention to additional
studies of the tradition.

She does not want to expose herself to worldly temptations:

> ich fürhte, solte ich werden alt,
> daz mich der werlte süeze
> zuhte under füeze,
> als sî vil manegen hât gezogen
> den ouch ir süeze hât betrogen.
> sô würde ich lîhte gote entsaget.   [700–705]

(I fear that if I should grow old worldly sweetness might drag me down as it has dragged very many who have been deceived by its sweetness. In that way I would easily deny God.)

Her fear is that she may renonunce God, and renounce Him for the same reasons that Heinrich had: to obtain *werlte süeze.*

The girl possesses the love of God, the *caritas* that Heinrich lacks.[6] Hartmann stresses her purity again and again.[7] For instance, it is said of her that in her love of Heinrich she looks after him *mit reiner kindes güete* (322), with the pure goodness of a child. For his part, *er dûhte sî vil reine* (344), he thought her very pure. So complete is her innocence that one might well compare her childlike goodness to the goodness of an angel, *der engel güete* (464–466). As she lies crying at the foot of her parents' bed, Hartmann notes that she bears the greatest goodness he has ever seen in a child (520–524). Her father and mother finally yield to her argument, and the pure girl, *diu reine maget* (903), rejoices. She approaches Heinrich and offers to sacrifice herself for him; deeply touched, he replies,

6 Willson, p. 527.
7 Fechter, p. 9.

ich erkenne dînen süezen muot,
din wille ist reine unde guot.   [937–938]

(I know your sweet purpose, your wish is pure and good.)

From the beginning, Heinrich recognizes that God has given her a sweet soul (348), that her purity must be attributed to Him. In time, he realizes further that he has failed to acknowledge his own debt to God:

dô nam ich sîn vil cleine war
der mir daz selbe wunschleben
von sînen gnâden hât gegeben.   [392–394]

(Then [before I became leprous] I took very little heed of Him who out of His mercy gave me that same perfect life.)

It remains for Heinrich to place himself in God's hands and accept his fate rather than renounce it.

His spiritual rebirth occurs at Salerno as the child is about to sacrifice herself. She is naked before the doctor but not ashamed because she is free of sin, in a state of innocence.[8] Heinrich peers through a crack in the wall and

---

[8] The girl's nudity has been interpreted in various ways. Arno Schirokauer, "Zur Interpretation des Armen Heinrich," *ZDA*, LXXXIII (1951–1952), 72–73, proposes that as she lies naked and bound, she is understood by Heinrich to be a martyr; it is not her beauty which moves him, but her moral significance. Willson, pp. 528–530, sees Christ-symbolism in the girl and stresses that her nudity signifies innocence. The idea of nudity as an expression of primal innocence has a long tradition. See George Boas, *Essays on Primitivism and Related Ideas in the Middle Ages* (New York, 1966), pp. 42-43; George Ferguson, *Signs and Symbols in Chris-*

sees her on the table. He compares his defiled body to her perfect one, and recognizes that his defilement is not merely physical:

> ir lîp der was vil wünneclich.
> nu sach er sî an unde sich
> und gewan ein niuwan muot:
> in dûhte dô daz niht guot,
> daz in dâ ê hâte,
> und verkêrte vil drâte
> sîn altez gemüete
> in eine niuwe güete.   [1233–1240]

(Her body was very delightful. Now he saw her and himself and assumed a new spirit. Then he thought that what he had formerly believed was not good, and he very quickly changed his old attitude into a new goodness.)

Her physical purity and beauty are signs of her spiritual purity, and Heinrich's recognition of this significance enables him to see his own physical condition as symbolic of his moral guilt. He perceives that since his need is for spiritual rather than physical cleansing, the girl's sacrifice is unnecessary as well as cruel, and so he prevents the operation. He is now able to accept God's omnipotence with humility: *gotes wille müeze an mir geschehen* (1276), What God wills for me must come to pass, he says. He has been put to a test as exacting as Job's; having purified him-

---

tian Art (New York, 1961), pp. 49–50. Leslie Sieffert, "The Maiden's Heart: Legend and Fairy-Tale in Hartmann's 'Der Arme Heinrich,' " *DVLG*, XXXVII (1963), 391–393, takes the nakedness as partly allegorical, partly erotic; in Heinrich's apprehension of her, there is "an element of appreciative love."

self spiritually, he is ready to be cleansed physically, to be made—like the girl—*reine unde wol gesunt*, pure and completely healthy (1360–1370). Accordingly, as with Job, Heinrich is healed by God and given more wealth and honor than before.[9] More profound than the increase in his wealth, however, is the change in his outlook. He can now be called *ein frumer ritter* (1340), a worthy, pious knight, for he knows that the source of honor lies in serving God, in doing honor to Him (1430–1436). His *übermuot* is tranformed into *ein niuwan muot*. Cured of his worldliness, Heinrich is cured of his leprosy.

Heinrich's moral failure, the result of his movement away from God and his commitment to the world, is the failure implicit in the idea of moral leprosy, as homiletic writing demonstrates. This failure underlies the significance of leprosy at nearly every appearance of it in literature. For example, in the legend of Constantine and Silvester, Constantine is typically presented as a worldly, unholy man. In a German version of the story, his leprosy is a punishment for his opposition to Christianity:

Ein keiser was zu Rome, der hiz Constantinus. Der was ein vient kristens glouben, und wo her kristine lute begreif daz liz her si toten. Der nachtes, do her lag uf sinem bette, do quam ein engel und brachte ein vaz mit wazzere und schut iz uf in, und her wart zu male uzsetzic.[10]

[9] For an examination of the Job-Heinrich parallels, see Fechter, pp. 2 ff.

[10] "Sanct Silvester: Tischrede aus dem Buch von der Heiligen Leben [1343–1349] von Hermann von Fritzlar," *Der Arme Heinrich Herrn Hartmanns von Aue und Zwei Jüngere Prosalegenden Verwandten Inhaltes*, ed. Wilhelm Wackernagel and Ernst Stadler (Basel, 1911), p. 171.

(In Rome, there was an emperor named Constantine. He was an enemy of the Christian faith, and wherever Christian people embraced it, he had them killed. One night, when he lay on his bed, an angel came and brought a vessel with water and tossed it on him, and he immediately became leprous.)

Although John Gower's rendering of the story in the *Confessio Amantis* (1390–1393)[11] does not make the cause of Constantine's leprosy explicit, it does imply that the disease is punitive. Saints Peter and Paul discuss Constantine's "wofull Soule" (3345) and tell him how Silvester had been forced to flee

> For drede of thee, which many a day
> Hast ben a fo to Cristes lay
> And hast destruid to mochel shame
> The prechours of his holy name.   [3353–3356]

(for fear of you, who for many a day have been a foe of Christ's law, and have destroyed—to your great shame —the preachers of His holy name.)

A Wyclifite text which compares Naaman and Constantine simply states, "Both these secular men were great lords and lepers."[12] And one of the damned in Dante's *Inferno* speaks of Constantine in terms which suggest that his leprosy was caused by pride:

[11] II. 3187–3496 in *The Complete Works of John Gower,* ed. G. C. Macaulay, II (Oxford, 1901).

[12] "The Clergy May Not Hold Property," *The English Works of Wyclif Hitherto Unprinted,* ed. F. D. Matthew, EETS, O.S., no. 74 (London, 1880), p. 377. According to the editor, the attribution of the work to Wyclif is uncertain.

Ma come Constantin chiese Silvestro
   d'entro Siratti a guerir della lebbra;
   così mi chiese questi per maestro
a guerir della sua superba febbra.   [XXVII.94–97]

(But as Constantine sought out Sylvester in Soracte to cure his leprosy, so this man [Pope Boniface VIII] sought me out as his physician to cure the fever of his pride.)[13]

According to the legend, Constantine learns that he can cure the disease by bathing in the blood of children, and so he requires that they be brought to his palace to be sacrificed for his health. However, at the last moment, he takes pity on them and sends them away, determined to continue as a leper rather than take innocent lives. The pity he shows pleases God, and Peter and Paul come to Constantine in a vision to tell him that Silvester can heal him. Constantine sends for Silvester, who cures the emperor by converting him to the Christian faith. In sum, the story of Constantine reveals the same structure as the tale of Heinrich and indeed of most stories in which a man is first punished by and then cured of leprosy: the leprosy chastizes the estrangement from God, and the submission to God brings about the cure. The story of the leper who is cured is typically the story of a redeemed sinner.

This pattern of movement away from and then back to God is repeated in nearly all versions of the Amis and Amiloun tale. The story is about two friends who are identical in appearance. One of them, Amis, finds himself in a

[13] *The Divine Comedy of Dante Alighieri,* trans. John D. Sinclair (New York, 1948), I, 338–339.

difficult position: he is accused of having made love to his overlord's daughter and his execution seems unavoidable. He is given the opportunity to prove his innocence in judicial combat, but since he is guilty of the accusation, the only possible consequence of the combat will be his death. However, his friend Amiloun agrees to undertake the battle for him, and the two men switch identities. Amis goes to Amiloun's wife and stays with her as her husband, though he carefully avoids committing adultery. Meanwhile, Amiloun fights the battle and vindicates Amis. In many of the versions, Amiloun, still posing as Amis, marries the daughter, but shortly afterward becomes a leper. His cure is brought about when Amis kills his two children so that Amiloun can bathe in their blood.

One study of the tale—by MacEdward Leach, in his edition of the middle English poem (late thirteenth century)[14] —proposes that the various renderings handle the material as either a romantic or a hagiographic story. In the group of hagiographic tales, the emphasis is on the saintliness of the pair and the miracles associated with them; the romantic versions stress the extraordinary friendship of the two knights.[15] It true enough that two of the romantic tales do

[14] *Amis and Amiloun*, EETS, O.S., no. 203 (London, 1937). All quotations of the Middle English poem are taken from this edition.

[15] The romantic stories exist in seven versions: a Latin poem by Radulfus Tortarius; an Anglo-Norman poem in three MSS, one of which is incomplete; a *chanson de geste;* the Middle English poem; a French miracle play; a Latin prose version in the *Historia Septem Sapientum Romae;* and a French poem which exists only in MS (and which Leach does not discuss). "The hagiographic versions are numerous; almost every language of Europe can furnish at least one." Detailed bibliographical references are given by Leach, pp. ix–xiv.

not have a religious orientation: "The *Seven Sages* account is wholly secular . . . . [the] leprosy is caused by poison" and "Radulfus Tortarius leaves the leprosy unmotivated."[16] The remaining versions are not taken to be devoid of all religious influence, but Leach does minimize the importance of that influence on them. He states that the English and Anglo-Norman tales are "Christian in background, not theme," and he allows that "the characters move in a Christian environment"; but he insists that the poems are not religious, do not aim at exalting Christian virtues, and are "fundamentally non-Christian." The three romantic versions which trace the cause of Amiloun's leprosy to bigamy give what "appears to be a 'tacked-on' explanation, a sophisticated one; and what is more important, it is a Christian explanation."[17] Leach is of course correct in showing that the romantic versions are not saints' lives and to that degree, at least, not Christian or religious in theme. So too is it valid—from the point of view of one interested in tracing the origins of a story—to distinguish between Christian ("tacked on") and non-Christian (original) elements, but it must be recognized that in four of the six romantic versions which Leach considers, Christian retellers of the tale were shaping a Christian story and entertaining a Christian audience. Perhaps their aim was not to write homilies, but a Christian ethic does inform the story, and so far as that is true, the Anglo-Norman, English, and French versions are fundamentally Christian.[18]

[16] *Amis and Amiloun*, pp. xxviii, lxiii.
[17] *Amis and Amiloun*, pp. xxii, xxv, xxvii.
[18] It has been suggested that the Middle English version is neither romance nor hagiography, but secular hagiography. See Ojars Kratins, "The Middle English *Amis and Amiloun*: Chivalric

The presence of a Christian point of view is perhaps nowhere more apparent than in the pivotal scene in which Amiloun is warned that he will become a leper. Leach's summary of the episode suggests that an unidentified voice from the sky warns Amiloun.[19] However, an angel is named as speaker in the Middle English poem, in the *chanson de geste*, and in the miracle play. In the Anglo-Norman variants, Amiloun is warned by a voice which is not named, but nevertheless the implication that the speaker is an angel is strong. In the Anglo-Norman *Amis e Amilun*, Amiloun and the girl, Flurie, are about to be married; they stand before the priest, who—according to tradition—asks that they give their names. Amiloun's problem is distinct, even if implicit: if he uses Amis' name he will profane the sacrament of marriage both by giving his name falsely and by committing bigamy; if he gives his own name, however, it will become obvious that Amis and Flurie committed the sin they were accused of. He must choose between the fidelity due God and the fidelity due his friend. As the priest demands his name, a voice warns Amiloun that if he marries

Romance or Secular Hagiography?" *PMLA*, LXXXI (1966), 347–354. Kratins correctly emphasizes the Christian influence on the poem, although his contention that the leprosy is not a punishment is open to question. William Calin's excellent study of the French *chanson de geste*, *Ami et Amile*, makes clear the importance of a Christian framework in that poem; his view is that Ami is divinely punished with leprosy for the crime of bigamy. See *The Epic Quest: Studies in Four Old French Chansons de Geste* (Baltimore, 1966), pp. 57–117, and especially pp. 89–90.

[19] "As the combat is about to begin, a voice comes out of the sky and warns him that if he fights this combat he will be punished with leprosy in three years (in some versions the voice gives this warning when he is about to marry the girl in his friend's name)" (p. xv).

the girl he will become a leper; he takes her because he
chooses not to betray Amis:

> Mais pur ceo ne vout lesser,
> Einz la receit com sa mulier.
> Ne voleit ke fust aparceu,
> Coment son frere sust deceu.   [719–722][20]

(Despite this he did not wish to stop, but took her as
his wife. He did not want it to be seen how his brother
had transgressed.)

The conflict between Amiloun's sacred and secular obligations is drawn clearly in one of the variant manuscripts.[21]
As he comes before the priest, Amiloun considers the alter-
natives. He declares to God his fear that he will never be
able to absolve himself of his sin if he refuses to give his
name; on the other hand, if he does admit his name he will
be accused by the king and will betray Flurie and Amis. At
this point the voice admonishes him, as if in reply to his
thoughts. In the Anglo-Norman variants, then, the warning is given in a decidedly religious context; there is every
probability that a divine injunction is delivered.

There is no doubt that in the French versions the admonition is given by an angel. According to the *chanson
de geste, Amis et Amiles,*

> Li cuens Amis ot fait son sairement,
> De vers le ciel vint uns angres volant,
> Desor l'espaule Amis de maintenant
> S'assist li angres.   [1806–1809][22]

---

[20] *Amis and Amiloun zugleich mit der altfranzösischen quelle,*
ed. Eugen Kölbing, *Altenglische Bibliothek,* II (Heilbronn, 1844),
153.

[21] Kölbing, pp. 152 f.

[22] *Amis et Amiles und Jourdains de Blaivies,* ed. Konrad Hofmann, 2d ed. (Erlangen, 1882), p. 90.

(Count Amis swore his oath. An angel came flying from the sky; now the angel seated himself on the shoulder of Amis.)

In the *Miracle de Nostre Dame d'Amis et d'Amille,* God sends Gabriel to tell Amis that

> il a sa foy mentie,
> Et que je vueil qu'il se chastie
> De tel affaire.   [1213–1215][23]

(he falsified his sworn word [*literally,* his faith], and that I declare that he chastize himself for this affair.)

Similarly, the English version is explicit that the voice delivers a divine warning:

> As he com prikand out of toun,
> Com a voice fram heuen adoun,
> Þat noman herd bot he,
> & sayd, "Þou kniȝt, sir Amiloun,
> God, þat suffred passioun,
> Sent þe bode bi me."   [1250–1254]

(As he came spurring out of town, a voice came down from heaven that no one heard but he, and said, "You knight, Sir Amiloun, God, who suffered passion, sends you a message through me.)

The difference between the English version and the other romantic versions is that in the latter, the warning is given as Amiloun, fraudulently presenting himself as Amis, is about to commit bigamy; in the former, the message comes as Amiloun, once again presenting himself as Amis, rides

---

[23] *Miracles de Nostre Dame par Personnages,* vol. IV, ed. Gaston Paris and Ulysse Robert, SATF (Paris, 1879), p. 44.

out to undertake judicial combat for his friend. The shift
in the time when the warning is given has been taken as a
shift in the significance of the leprosy. Kratins argues that,
whereas in the other versions the leprosy is a punishment
for bigamy, in the English version it is no punishment at
all: "It is a visitation of divine grace with the goal of verify-
ing, before the tale is over, that both friends in the severest
of trials 'trew weren in al þing,' as the poem states at the
outset."[24] No one will fail to admit that the story gives
Amis and Amiloun the chance to prove their loyalty to one
another, but although the leprosy is a test of loyalty, it is
at the same time a punishment. The warning calls upon
Amiloun to assign priorities to his loyalties and being
stricken with the disease is a chastisement for the choice
he makes.

The voice from heaven speaks to Amiloun as he is about
to do battle for Amis. It tells him:

> "ȝif þou þis bataile vnderfong,
> Þou schalt haue an euentour strong
> Wiþ-in þis ȝeres þre;
> & or þis þre ȝere ben al gon,
> Fouler mesel nas neuer non
> In þe world, þan þou schal be!"   [1255–1260]

> (If you undertake this battle, you shall experience a
> severe adventure within three years; before these three
> years are gone, there will not be a fouler leper in the
> world than you shall be.)

The clear implication is that Amiloun will become leprous
if he poses as Amis at the trial by combat; the fact that
there may be no other character in medieval literature who

---

[24] Kratins, p. 351.

is punished for practicing deception at a judicial ordeal[25] does not alter the fact that Amiloun is punished for his deception. Yet Kratins proposes that *Amis and Amiloun* does not deviate from the traditional presentation of the tricked ordeal: the "euentour" which the angel prophesies is not a punishment (the voice makes "a morally neutral statement"[26]) but a test of Amiloun's fidelity to Amis. There is no question that Amiloun's fidelity is being tested —but the test is not limited to Amiloun's fidelity to his friend. His fidelity to God is tested as well.

Before the fight, Amiloun swears an oath before God that he never kissed the girl (1285–1296). According to the convention of the judicial combat, God lets truth govern the outcome—but the God in *Amis and Amiloun* does not let the results be limited by the idea of literal truth. Although Amiloun did not kiss the girl, he is not the man he pretends to be. Hence, although Amiloun is permitted to win the combat, he is punished for the deception he practices by giving a false statement under oath. In short, when the voice from heaven speaks, it offers Amiloun the choice of being true to God and seeing his friend die, or being untrue to God (by dishonoring the oath sworn before Him) and seeing his friend live.

Significantly, the hagiographic versions emphasize the identical conflict between sacred and secular obligations, though admittedly the punishment with leprosy follows the bigamous marriage. Still, before the combat, Amicus considers the implication of what he is about to do:

Heu michi, qui mortem huius comitis tam fraudulenter cupio! Scio enim, quod si illum interfecero, reus ero ante supernum

[25] Leach, *Amis and Amiloun*, pp. lxxxvi, lxiv.
[26] Kratins, p. 351.

judicem, si vero meam vitam tulerit, de me semper obprobrium narrabitur perpetuum.

(O, woe is me, who so desire the death of this steward through a trick! I know truly that if I kill him I will be arraigned before the celestial judge; if truly he should take my life, I will always be held in complete disgrace.)

He knows that if he kills Ardericus, God will judge him guilty. Amicus, who must decide whether he wishes to be condemned by the world or by God, remains loyal to his friend, kills Ardericus, and is awarded the girl. Of course, his loyalty and self-sacrifice are heroic, and the hero cannot be damned for so admirable a fault. Therefore, God extends his grace to Amicus, who will receive salvation. But first he must be purged of his sin, and accordingly God strikes him with leprosy: "Amicum . . . percussit Deus morbo lepre," in keeping with what is written in the Bible: "juxta illud quod scriptum est: Omnem filium, quem Deus recipit, corripit, flagellat, et castigat."[27] "Every son

---

[27] Kölbing, pp. ciii–civ. At least three readers of this passage have interpreted it as evidence that the leprosy is not a punishment but a sign of God's love (see Calin, pp. 88 f.; Jessie Crossland, *The Old French Epic* [Oxford, 1951], p. 222; and Kratins, p. 350). However, both the full sense of the passage (with the verbs *percutio, corripio, flagello,* and *castigo*) and the biblical passage alluded to suggest that the leprosy is simultaneously a consequence of divine love and displeasure. The Scripture is Paul's Epistle to the Hebrews, 12:6, in which he reminds them of Proverbs 3:11–12: "quem enim diligit dominus castigat flagellat autem omnem filium quem recipit." "For whom the Lord loveth, he chastiseth; and he scourgeth every son whom he receiveth." Paul's message is that God's scourging is a form of paternal rebuke and correction: "in disciplina perseverate tamquam filiis uobis offert se deus. Quis enim filius quem non corripit pater." "Persevere under discipline. God

whom God receives, He chides, scourges, and chastises."
"Dex chostoie celui cui il aime."[28] "God punishes the one
He loves"—as a stern father punishes a disobedient child.
The moral context in the hagiographic versions is thus
echoed in the Middle English poem: in both, a man knows
that he will displease God by compromising truth.

The transgression was not taken as a minor one. The
medieval preachers saw fraudulence as a form of moral
leprosy, and Dante locates the fradulent in the eighth circle
of hell, where the worst sins are punished. The last group
in Malebolge, the pit of iniquity, are the falsifiers, who are
punished with innumerable diseases. Here, where the
damned are mutilated, where their limbs are putrid, Dante
sees two who were alchemists, falsifiers of metals. They
are spotted with scabs from head to foot and must scratch
perpetually,

> per la gran rabbia
> del pizzicor, che non ha piu soccorso.   [XXXIX.80–81]

(for the great fury of their itch that has no other
relief.)[29]

These two are lepers, who suffer the usual torments of the
disease, but suffer them unceasingly. Like all those in
Malebolge, like all sinners and thus like all moral lepers,
they are damned for having moved away from God, as
their position near the very center of Hell implies.

Amiloun fully recognizes the nature of his predicament.

---

dealeth with you as with his sons; for what son is there, whom
the father does not correct?" (12:7).

[28] *Amis et Amile*, in *Nouvelles françoises en prose du XIIIe siècle*, ed. L. Moland and C. D'Héricault (Paris, 1856), p. 60.

[29] *The Divine Comedy of Dante Alighieri*, I, 362–363.

After the warning is delivered, he considers all the possi-
bilities—whether

> To flen, oþer to fiȝting gon;
> In hert him liked ille.
> He þouȝt, "ȝif y beknowe mi name,
> Þan schal mi broþor go to schame,
> Wiþ sorwe þai schul him spille."   [1277–1281]

> (to flee, or to go fighting; in his heart, neither appealed
> to him. He thought, "if I reveal my name, then my
> brother shall be shamed, they shall destroy him, with
> sorrow.")

To flee would be to break his troth with Amis, to engage
in battle would be to swear an oath deceitfully. Only a man
who knows that fraudulence is sinful would hesitate, and
only that kind of man would consider that he ought to
reveal his name. Obviously, whatever the poet's reason for
eliminating the bigamous marriage from the poem, it was
not to relieve Amiloun of moral guilt.[30] Indeed, the leprosy
is a symbol of that guilt.

The nature of Amiloun's transgression is emphasized by
the act that Amis must perform to heal him of leprosy.
Just as Amiloun was given a divine message, so also is Amis.
An angel comes to him as he sleeps and tells him that to
cure Amiloun, Amis' two children must be killed and
Amiloun bathed in their blood. By this means,

[30] One ought at least to consider the possibility that the poet
felt the bigamous marriage added little or nothing to Amiloun's
guilt. When, in other versions, Amiloun gives Amis' name at the
marriage ceremony, he is simply repeating the deception he had
practiced at the judicial combat; the sole difference is that at the
marriage he states he is Amis, whereas at the combat he lets everyone assume he is.

Þurch godes grace, þat is so gode,
His wo schuld wende oway.   [2207–2208]

(Through the grace of God, that is so good, his woe
shall go away.)

Notice that the circumstances surrounding the second
message from heaven are very different from those encountered earlier.[31] In Amiloun's case, the voice speaks to
him only after he has decided to ride out to do battle. It
does not propose a course of action but warns against one
in terms which promise the living death of the pariah (1261–
1272). In the second case, the angel offers a cure, a promise
of rebirth sanctioned by God. To be sure, the choice is a
hard one—no man who loves his children kills them easily,
and Amis naturally considers that to kill them would be to
commit a deadly sin (2245–2247)—but the angel gives no
suggestion that Amis would place his soul in jeopardy. If
anything, the angel suggests that by sacrificing the children
he would be accomplishing the will of God. Amis recognizes this fact. When he tells his wife what he has done,
he says:

"Be bliþe & glad of mode;
For bi him þat þis warld wan
Boþe mi childer ich haue slan."   [2379–2381]

("Be happy and glad of manner; for by virtue of Him
who rescued this world, I have slain both my children.")

Accordingly, the choice offered Amis is the reverse of the

[31] Cf. Kratins, p. 353: "The two sacrifices, being part of the
same theme of *trewþe,* are made as much as possible parallel."

one given Amiloun. Where it is suggested to Amiloun that
if he compromises a sworn oath God will strike him with
leprosy, Amis is told that if he bows his will to God's, God
will remove that leprosy. In sacrificing his children, then,
Amis demonstrates his *trewþe* with Amiloun and with
God. There is no doubt in his case, at least, that he was
"trew in al þing" (34).

But what of Amiloun? Can it validly be said of him, as
the poem indeed has it (34–36, 2506–2508), that he was
perfect in his *trewþe?* Kratin's suggestion that the leprosy
is not a punishment for a failure in *trewþe* has the attractive-
ness of eliminating what otherwise seems an inconsistency,
but it has the limitation of disregarding what the poem
establishes firmly, if implicitly: the leprosy is a consequence of the judicial battle, and a punishment for the
deceit which Amiloun practices. Secondly, the inconsistency is only apparent. Amiloun's lapse in faith is no more
than momentary. The faith he owes God comes into conflict with the faith due Amis, and to be firm in one he must
slight the other. Moreover, he knows that he must be punished, and he accepts what God metes out to him:

> "Certes," he seyd, "for drede of care
> To hold mi treuþe schal y nouȝt spare,
> Lete god don alle his wille." [1282–1284]

> ("Certainly," he said, "for fear of suffering I shall not
> cease to be steadfast—let God do all His will.")

To be sure, "reduced to a mere nothing, he accepts his
affliction as a blessing. Since it is a consequence of his
trewþe to Amis, Amiloun never in all his wanderings as a

beggar rebels against his lot, just as a saint never rebels against the suffering imposed on him for the sake of his faith."[32] From the beginning, Amiloun accepts his punishment with humility and faith in God.

The nature of Amiloun's perfection is revealed when he is compared to Hartmann von Aue's Heinrich. Heinrich, a proud and worldly man, is punished for his sinful way of life, not for a sinful act; Amiloun is punished because he sins at one moment in time, when—given the choice—he elects to place his fidelity to Amis before his fidelity to God. However, even while sinning against God, Amiloun submits to Him: "Let God do all His will," he says (1284). Amiloun enters into sin consciously, with full awareness that he is sacrificing himself for his friend; in contrast to Heinrich, he is not self-seeking or blind to his religious obligations.

Amiloun's sinfulness is not as intense as Heinrich's, and consequently Amiloun's leprosy is not healed in the way Heinrich's is. Amiloun sins, is punished with the disease, and pays for his transgression through his suffering. Because the angel tells him that his illness will be his punishment, he knows its import from the moment it strikes him. The cure of Amiloun's leprosy therefore does not depend upon a recognition of and repentance for his sinfulness. Unlike Heinrich, he can remain passive while his cure is obtained. It is fitting that Amis should be required to act in order to bring about the cure of his friend; if Amiloun sacrificed himself in order to save Amis, it is right that Amis should make a personal sacrifice to save Amiloun. Amiloun, who has already done more than could reason-

[32] Kratins, p. 353.

ably be required of any man, need do nothing to obtain his cure. His release from leprosy does not depend upon a spiritual transformation but upon a ritual act: Amis must sacrifice his children and bathe Amiloun in their innocent blood.

On the other hand, for Heinrich, a spiritual reformation does eliminate the leprosy. Although the doctor tells Heinrich that a virgin's blood could cure him, the fact is that the cure is obtained when Heinrich achieves the humility and patience which Amiloun has all along. When Heinrich obtains the insight which Amiloun has at the outset, when he says, "What God wills for me must come to pass!" (1276), his leprosy can be taken from him. Heinrich's leprosy is the mark of a sinfulness far more profound than Amiloun's, and its cure accordingly depends upon a spiritual awakening. In contrast, Amiloun is at all times aware of the state of his soul. He is an exemplary figure with a human flaw, a flaw he atones for through his suffering, and surely no one who hears of him feels that the bliss of heaven that God grants him for his "trewþe and godhede" (2506) is undeserved.

In brief, the role of leprosy in the Middle English *Amis and Amiloun* is not essentially different from its role in most other versions of the story, whether romantic or hagiographic. For the most part, the story associates the leprosy with deceit, and it makes the association in a religious context. The deceit is practiced in conscious disregard of divine power, and the punishment for the sin is therefore divinely ordered.

The often repeated pattern of offense against divine authority and consequent chastisement is found again in *The Testament of Cresseid*, by Robert Henryson (died before 1508). The poet calls his work a "tragedie" (4),[33] and a tragedy it is as that form was understood during the Middle Ages: it traces the fall of a person of high position from happiness to misery. At the same time, the poem reveals a moral structure which gives meaning to the tragic outline of the plot. The heroine is the cause of her own downfall, not an innocent victim of arbitrary fortune. She sins, and because she sins she is punished by the gods[34] with leprosy.

The poem is a sequel to Chaucer's *Troilus and Criseyde;* the story begins after Cresseid has left Troilus for Diomed, and after Diomed has in turn deserted her. Cresseid is still a beautiful woman and still a person of rank, but the corruption of her soul which culminates in the corruption of her body is already under way—has indeed been under way for some time. She is sensuous and worldly, one who delights in her wanton bower and bed, in spices and wine, cups of gold and silver, sauces, meats, garments, gardens, fame, and honor (416–437). But more than anything, she is a lustful woman. Diomed, we are told,

> had all his appetyte,
> And mair, fulfillit of this fair ladie.   [71–72]

[33] All quotations of the *Testament* are from the edition by Denton Fox (London, 1968). Quotations are followed by line numbers in brackets or parentheses. Fox's edition provides an excellent discussion of the poem and its backgrounds. Much of my discussion corroborates information presented in his book.

[34] The gods in Henryson's poem are Cupid and the pagan deities associated with each of the planets. Nonetheless, they "belong to the theological code and when Cresseid offends against them she offends against God's holy laws." See E. M. W. Tillyard, "Henryson: *The Testament of Cresseid*, 1470?" in *Five Poems: 1470–1870* (London, 1948), p. 16. Cf. Sydney Harth, "Henryson Reinterpreted," *EIC*, XI (1961), 471–480.

(had all his appetite, and more, satisfied by this fair lady.)

Now, rejected by her lover, she walks "into the Court, commoun" (77), that is, she becomes a whore. Henryson's apostrophe to Cresseid emphasizes the tragedy of it:

> O fair Creisseid, the flour and A per se
> Of Troy and Grece, how was thow fortunait
> To change in filth all thy feminitie,
> And be with fleschelie lust sa maculait,
> And go amang the Greikis air and lait,
> Sa giglotlike takand thy foull plesance!
> I haue pietie thow suld fall sic mischance!   [78–84]

(O fair Cresseid, the flower and paragon of Troy and Greece, how evil was your fortune to change all your femininity into filth, and be so spotted with fleshly lust, and go so like a harlot among the Greeks, early and late, taking your foul enjoyment! I have pity that you should come in for such mischance!)

She is spotted by her sexuality, *maculait*, says Henryson, and his word looks forward to the macules of leprosy which ultimately make her hideous and signify her moral condition.

Cresseid presumes to blame the false Cupid and his blind mother, Venus, for the fact that she is "fra luifferis left, and all forlane" (140), deserted and violated by her lovers.[35] She angrily abuses the two gods, voicing her re-

---

[35] H. Harvey Wood, *The Poems and Fables of Robert Henryson*, 2d ed. (Edinburgh, 1958), p. 145, observes that the meaning of *forlane* in this line is ambiguous. It signifies either forsaken or deflowered, prostituted, violated. The ambiguity may well be intentional; in any case, there is little justification for preferring

gret that she ever worshiped them and claiming that they misled her and caused her to be rejected (124–141). Cupid is incensed that she should trace her infelicity and unclean and lecherous living to the gods. She blasphemes his name and slanders and defames Venus. "Was neuer to goddes done sic violence" (292), he says, and demands revenge. His request is granted. Cresseid offends love and the gods, and according to the traditional pattern she is castigated with leprosy. Saturn and Cynthia, the goddess of the Moon,[36] decree that she shall suffer pain and torment, an incurable sickness, and be abominable to all lovers (302–308); her insolence, play, and wantonness shall be changed to great disease (319–320).

Henryson makes the terrible justice of the punishment clear. Cresseid is proud and worldly. She rebukes the very gods she should have thanked for whatever happiness they saw fit to grant her. For her pride, the gods humiliate her, much as Hartmann's Heinrich was humiliated—they strike her with the disease which most effectively destroys her arrogance. The one who was insolent before the gods is made to go begging from people who abhor her: "Quhair thow cummis, ilk man sall fle the place"—Where you come, each man shall flee the place, says Cynthia (341).

In addition, Cresseid's leprosy is a particularly suitable

---

the first meaning, as Wood does. Both Cresseid's career and Cupid's rebuke of her support the second sense of the word, and that sense is in keeping with Henryson's emphasis of her unchastity. Cf. Fox, p. 96 (note to line 140).

[36] For the relationship of Cresseid's leprosy to astrology, see Marshall W. Stearns, "Robert Henryson and the Leper Cresseid," *MLN*, LIX (1944), 265–269; Johnstone Parr, "Cresseid's Leprosy Again," *MLN*, LX (1945), 487–491.

punishment for her promiscuity. Not only does it ravage her beauty, but what is more, because leprosy was commonly understood to be a venereal disease, a consequence of lust, it makes her past sinfulness apparent to her and to all who see her. The nature of the malady brings home to Cresseid the justice of what the gods do to her. She recognizes that her sickness is the result of her lechery, not the gods' capriciousness. "Sa [efflated] I was in wantones" (549), she admits, so puffed out in wantonness.

> "My mynd in fleschelie foull affectioun
> Was inclynit to lustis lecherous:
> Fy fals Cresseid; O trew knicht Troylus!"   [558–560]

> ("My mind, with foul fleshly leaning, was ever inclined to lecherous lusts: Fie, false Cresseid; O, true knight Troilus!")

Thus Cresseid sees the moral structure which underlies the suffering she undergoes and finally attaches the blame for her condition to herself. She accepts the responsibility for what her leprosy punishes and symbolizes: her pride and her lust.

Cresseid is not the only figure in medieval literature whose leprosy is attached to debauchery. In a poem by Rutebeuf (ca. 1225–1280), "La Disputaison de Charlot et du Barbier," one of the figures—the barber—is described as a leper.[37] The barber's antagonist, Charlot, says that Saint Lazarus has struck the barber in the face with an ulcer (17–22); he has a leprous visage:

[37] *Oeuvres complètes de Rutebeuf*, ed. Edmond Faral and Julia Bastin, II (Paris, 1960), 260–265. Line references to the poem are given in parentheses or brackets.

"Barbier, or vienent les groiseles,
Li groiselier sont boutone;
Et je vous raport les noveles
Qu'el front vous sont li borjon ne.
Ne sai se ce seront ceneles
Qui ce vis ont avirone;
Els seront vermeilles et beles
Avant que l'en ait moissone."   [65–72]

("Barber, the currants come, the currant bushes have
budded; and I tell you the news that your forehead has
grown buds. I do not know if these buds which have
surrounded your face will be scarlet holly berries;
they'll be crimson and beautiful before they're har-
vested.")

The barber knows that the nodules on his face are leprous,
and his response—"Ce n'est mie meselerie" (73), It's not
leprosy—suggests the accuracy of Charlot's diagnosis.

The barber's disease is appropriate in a man of his pro-
fession. He is not, after all, a barber. He has neither razor
nor scissor, indeed no implements whatsoever, and in any
event he does not know how to cut hair or shave (33–36).
Still, he does perform certain services. Charlot calls him
"va li dire" (56), a procurer of women, and Rutebeuf
verifies that he does his work well:

Li Barbiers connoist bone gent
Et si les sert et les honeure
Et met en els cors et argent,
Paine de servir d'eure en eure.   [97–100]

(The barber knows good people, and also serves and
honors them, and spends heart and money on them,
labors to serve from hour to hour.)

By coupling comments on the barber's expertise and physical appearance, Rutebeuf suggests that the leprosy and
the pandering are linked to each other:

> Et set son mestier bel et gent
> Se besoins li recoroit seure;
> Et s'a en lui molt biau sergent,
> Que, com plus vit, et plus coleure.   [101–104]

> (And he does his work well and nobly, if the need
> should come upon him; and he has the look of a pretty
> boy indeed, for the more he lives, the more his face
> reddens.)

Underlying Rutebeuf's poem is the common idea that leprosy and carnality go hand in hand.

The strength of the connection between the two gave
the malady a moral significance which is strikingly demonstrated in the legend of Tristan and Isolde. In the versions
of the legend by Eilhart von Oberge and Béroul, the adul-
terous lovers are sentenced to burn for their act. Tristan
manages to escape, but Isolde is led to the stake. At the last
moment, a group of lepers appears and their spokesman
proposes that she be turned over to them; he has a punishment, he suggests, which will fit the crime more perfectly
than Mark's. The leper in Eilhart's *Tristram und Isalde*
(ca. 1170–1180)[38] is blunt in his advice to Mark. Isolde
must die dishonorably, but death by fire is not dishonor-
able enough.

> einen tôd wil ich dir nennen
> dâ von sie mêr lasters habete.   [4270–4271]

[38] Ed. Franz Lichenstein, *Eilhart von Oberge*, QFSK, vol. XIX
(Strassburg, 1877).

("I will name you a death by which she will have more shame.")

Let the lepers have her in common:

> dô sprach der herzoge, ich wil sie
> mînen sîchen bringen:
> die suln sie alle minnen,
> sô stirbet sie lesterlîchen.   [4276–4279]

(The duke spoke: "I will bring her to my sick ones: they shall all love her, so that she will die dishonorably.")

Clearly, the appeal of the punishment is its awesome humiliation and the fact that it matches the crime; Isolde lived by passion, let her die by passion.

In Béroul's version (ca. 1160–1170),[39] the leper Ivain explains his reasons for wanting to dispose of Isolde. It is not simply that he can offer Mark a more fitting punishment than burning, but also that Mark can meet a need of his:

> "Veez, j'ai ci conpaignons cent;
> Yseut nos done, s'ert conmune;
> Paior fin dame n'ot mais une.
> Sire, en nos a si grant ardor
> Soz ciel n'a dame qui un jour
> Peüst sofrir nostre convers."   [1192–1197]

("See, I have here one-hundred companions; give Isolde to us, and she will be held in common. Never will a woman have a worse end. Sire, there is in us such great ardor that there is not a woman on earth who could endure our intercourse for one day.")

[39] *The Romance of Tristran by Beroul: A Poem of the Twelfth Century,* ed. A Ewert (Oxford, 1939).

Béroul's characterization of the band of lepers is an example in poetry of an idea which permeates medieval culture. Ivain's words echo Aretaeus' comment that the leper is tormented by an "irresistible and shameless impulse *ad coitum*" and they also find their analogue in the bestiality depicted in *Jaufré*, a thirteenth-century Provencal Arthurian romance.[40] The hero of the poem, Jaufré, is approached by a woman who asks him to rescue her child. The infant has been abducted by a leper, who wants to obtain blood in order to cure the disease. Jaufré follows the leper, who enters a building; when Jaufré goes in after him, the first thing he sees is a leper on a bed with a beautiful young girl:

> E us mezels fers e estrains
> Jai en un leit, e tenc lunc se
> Una piusela, qe nun cre
> Qe el mun n'aja belasor,
> Car pus ac fresca la color
> Qe rosa, cant es ades nada,
> E fu sa gonela esquintada
> Tro aval desos la tetina
> Qe ac pus blanca qe farina.
> E plais fort e menet gran dol,
> E ac pus grosses qe no sol
> Amdos los oils, tant ac plorat.   [2298–2309][41]

(And another leper, fierce and strange, was lying on a bed and embracing a maiden whom I believe had no equal in beauty in the world. She had a complexion more fresh than a rose just opened, and her tunic was torn open as far as below her breasts, which were more

[40] See Paul Remy, pp. 208–210.

[41] *Jaufré: Roman arthurien du XIIIe siècle en vers provençaux*, ed. Clovis Brunel, SATF (Paris, 1943), I, 82.

white than flour. She was weeeping violently and ex-
hibiting great grief, and she had cried so much that
both eyes were swollen.)

The beautiful girl is clearly no more than a sexual object
to the vicious leper, who is unmoved by her protestations.
When interrupted by Jaufré, he is about to satisfy the great
passion which Béroul's Ivain suggests is natural to lepers.
Ivain asks for Isolde precisely because she can satisfy that
passion, and he persuades Mark to turn her over to his band
of lepers by promising that if she lives with them, she will
come to acknowledge the illicit nature of her own lust:

> Donc savra bien Yseut la givre
> Que malement avra ovre.   [1214–1215]

> (Hence, Isolde the serpent will know well that she be-
> haved evilly.)

Mark recognizes the appropriateness of the punishment
and releases Isolde to the lepers: the adulteress driven by
base sexual passion must now satisfy the even more base,
more animal desires of Ivain and his company.

The licentious nature of Isolde's passion is indicated by
the punishment intended for her. Similarly, Tristan's lust
is signified by the leper's disguise he assumes in the version
by Thomas of Britain (after 1155–ca. 1170). Tristan, who
has been separated from Isolde, is driven by his love to see
her, but because he cannot risk being recognized by Mark,
he must conceal his identity. He dresses himself in ragged
clothing and by means of an herb he makes his face puffed
and swollen like a leper's. Of course, from one point of
view, his disguise is nothing more than a means of allowing him to gain entrance to the court, since his deformed

face is unrecognizable. In the story of Wistasse the monk, Wistasse also disguises himself as a leper and equips himself with the implements lepers carried—and all this solely in order to deceive and mock his enemies.[42] However, Tristan's disguise serves a purpose beyond that of allowing him to approach the court and beg without arousing suspicion. It is made clear that Tristan was greatly overcome by love —"Mult fud Tristran suspris d'amur" (1773).[43] He comes to Isolde as her paramour, and his appearance and his supplication permit him to announce to her his need as her lover:

> Tristran la veit, del sun li prie,
> Mais Ysolt nel reconnut mie;
> Il vait après e si flavele,
> A halte vuiz vers li apele,
> Del sun requert, per Deu amur,
> Pitusement, par grant tendrur.   [1801–1806]

(Tristan sees her and begs a gift of her, but Ysolt does not recognize him. He follows her, clacking, and loudly calls to her, appealing to her piteously by the love of God for alms in a most heart-rending way.)

The gift that Tristan seeks is not alms, it is love, and when Isolde finally recognizes him, what she tries to give him is not alms but her ring, the symbol of her love.

A similar scene is found in Eilhart's version of the story,

---

[42] *Wistasse le Moine: Altfranzösischer Abenteuerroman des XIII. Jahrhunderts*, ed. Wendelin Foerster and Johann Trost (Halle, 1891), ll. 1398–1491.

[43] *Le Roman de Tristan par Thomas*, ed. Joseph Bedier, SATF, I (Paris, 1902). The translation here and below is by A. T. Hatto, *Gottfried von Strassburg, Tristan . . . with the surviving fragments of the Tristran of Thomas* (Baltimore, 1960), p. 332.

though his account is briefer than Thomas' and differs in some important details.[44] For instance, in Thomas' version, Brangane—who despises Tristan because she has been shamed through him—does not permit Isolde to give her ring to Tristan; in Eilhart's poem, it is not Brangane but Isolde who will have nothing to do with Tristan. In order to reconcile himself with her, he approaches her in his leper disguise, pleading for recognition, but in her anger she has him driven away (7026–7048). Thus, the circumstances in the two poems are unalike, but the symbolism of the leper is the same: in both versions Tristan is the lover in need, the adulterer driven by his sexual passion.

Tristan appears disguised as a leper in Béroul as well, where the incident differs from the episodes in both Eilhart and Thomas. Isolde, who is called upon to prove that she is not an adulteress, must undergo a judicial ordeal; if she can carry a hot iron in her hands without burning herself, she will be declared innocent. In order to succeed at the ordeal, she sends word to Tristan to appear in the guise of a leper. Tristan follows her directions, arrives, and in the manner of a leper begs from those present. He seeks alms from Mark, and in the ensuing conversation the symbolism of the leprosy is clearly drawn. Mark asks Tristan how long he has been a leper. Tristan replies that he has been diseased for three years and that he became ill through his lover:

"Sire, trois anz i a, ne ment.
Tant con je fui en saine vie,

[44] Pierre Jonin, *Les Personnages féminins dans les romans français de Tristan au XIIe siècle: Étude des influences contemporaines*, Publication des annales de la faculté des lettres, Aix-en-Provence, new series, no. 22 (Gap, 1958), pp. 39–41.

Molt avoie cortoise amie,
Por lié ai je ces boces lees."   [3760–3763]

("Sire, three years, I do not lie. As long as I was in
good health I had a gracious lover. Because of her I
have these large swellings.")

His answer can be taken in two ways. On one level he
speaks as a leper suffering from venereal disease; on the
other level he speaks as the lover who three years before
shared the love potion with Isolde. Mark does not perceive
the ambiguity and he presses the leper for details; he must
know how the woman gave him the disease. Tristan replies:

"Dans rois, ses sires ert meseaus,
O lié faisoie mes joiaus,
Cist maus me prist de la comune.
Mais plus bele ne fu que une.
"Qui est ele?" "La bele Yseut;
Einsi se vest con cele seut."   [3771–3776]

("Sir king, her lord was a leper, I took my pleasure
with her, and as a result of the intercourse, I caught
the disease. But only one woman surpasses her beauty."
"Who is she?" "The beautiful Isolde; she dresses just as
she [the woman who gave me leprosy] does.")

The answer Mark receives is a reasonable explanation: the
physicians held that one mode of contagion involved intercourse with a woman shortly after she had relations with
a leper. What Mark does not understand is that Tristan's
reply equates the woman of the story with Isolde and her
leprous lord with Mark. It is Tristan's intention to insult
Mark, to mock his cuckoldry, to tell him that they have
both been sleeping with the same woman. Later, Isolde

takes advantage of Tristan's disguise in a similar way. When she arrives for the ordeal, she has the leper carry her over water on his back so that she can swear truthfully that there was never a man between her thighs but the leper and Mark (3882–3986, 4189–4231). Tristan's feigned leprosy, then, is manifestly a symbol of his adultery and his passion.

Ulrich von Lichtenstein uses the same symbol in his *Frauendienst* (1255).[45] In his poem, Ulrich tells how he served a woman because of his undying love for her. The relationship between Ulrich and his lady has the outward forms of a proper affair of courtly love: the woman is married, Ulrich abases himself in her service, and she is aloof, demanding, and unreachable. The consequence of this situation is that Ulrich must do extravagant things to please his lady (he has his little finger cut off and sent to her, for instance), but it appears that nothing he does will earn him the final reward he seeks—sexual intercouse. Ulrich leads a frustrated life.

On one occasion, after she receives a love lyric from Ulrich, the woman sends for him. Because she does not want their relationship to be discovered, she instructs him to come disguised as a leper and, in addition, makes it clear to him that she will not consent to have sexual intercourse. What she does is to clothe him in the garments of his lust and his humiliation, for it is her purpose to mock and degrade him. However, he hopefully does what the woman requires him to. He arrives at her castle on a Sunday morn-

[45] *Ulrich's von Liechtenstein Frauendienst*, ed. Reinhold Bechstein (Leipzig, 1888), II, 34–84 (strophes 1101–1284). In additional references to the poem, the numbers in parentheses or brackets represent the strophes in which the quoted lines are contained.

ing and joins the band of lepers who sit begging before it. According to a prearranged plan, Ulrich has his presence announced to his lady, who requires him to wait until evening, when he will be told why he has been sent for. Obediently, Ulrich goes back to the lepers, who are filthy and mutilated, and he suffers the indignity of having to eat with them. When evening comes, he is told to wait until morning. Ulrich complains but does as directed. He eats again with the lepers, sleeps in a field, is rained on, bitten by worms, vermin, and insects, and nearly frozen to death. Morning comes, but once again Ulrich is told to be patient and continue in his diguise until that evening, when he returns and is told to wait until nightfall. After sunset, Ulrich comes back to the castle and hides in a ditch. While he is there, the head steward of the castle stands over him and urinates on him. But finally he receives the signal to come to his lady. He takes off his dirtied clothes, and after some trouble succeeds in being lifted to a balcony and given fresh clothing. Ulrich is now close to receiving the reward he hopes for, and he is brought to the woman, who sits beautifully clothed on a sofa—in the presence of eight other women. Ulrich comments that their presence is a vexation. The cause of his annoyance is apparent: how can he have sexual intercourse with eight women looking on? Nonetheless, he kneels before the lady and asks for his reward:

> "sol ich iu hie geligen bî
> so bin ich alles des gewert,
> des mîn lîp ie ze vreuden gert.
> iwer gewern mac mir hie geben
> hôhen muot und werdez leben

immer mêr gar al mîn zît:
ir sît, an der mîn freude lît."   [1206]

("If I should lie here next to you, then I am bestowed with all that my person [*or,* body] ever desired for joy. Your bestowal can give me spiritual exaltation and worthy life for ever more, fully for all my life: you are the one in whom my joy resides.")

Ulrich's demand is understandable, but coarse, and in any case he has been told that the lady will not consider taking him as her sexual partner. She tells him as much again, and explains that she has brought him to the castle simply in order to honor him for his service. Ulrich is dismayed, and he protests, but to no avail. Still, the lady prolongs his hope by assuring him that if he does her will, she will do his. She directs him to get into a sheet suspended from a balcony; he will be let down and then pulled up in it; when he is retrieved, she tells him, she will welcome him. Ulrich climbs into the sheet and is let down a little. As he holds her hand, she takes him by the chin and says, "friunt, nu küsse mich!" (1268), Friend, now kiss me! Joyously, he lets go her hand—and she lets him fall to earth.

The episode is farcical. Ulrich tries to live according to an idea of love which should exalt the lover and refine him, but he is a common sensual man with common, sensual desires, and none of his posturing, his pleading on bended knee, his talk of his *hoher muot*, spiritual exaltation, succeeds in masking his carnality. Ulrich is not exalted, but debased, as his experience in the ditch or his descent from the balcony ought to remind him. Further, Ulrich's leper's disguise does not hide his real identity. Rather, as a symbol of his coarse lust, his frustrated sexual passion, it reveals his true nature.

It is the symbolic use of leprosy in *Frauendienst,* not the devices of the plot, which recalls the use of the leprosy disguise in the Tristan legend. In *Frauendienst,* the episode has two parts: first the man disguises himself as a leper at the direction of his lady, and then he is comically ridiculed and rejected by her. None of the Tristan versions that we have examined agrees exactly with this outline, nor indeed does any one of the Tristan versions agree completely with any other. However, all the episodes containing the disguise motif do share one important characteristic: in each, the true inner nature of the man is revealed by the disguise he wears. The inner lust is shown by the outer corruption.

The use of leprosy as a disguise in *Frauendienst* and the Tristan story differs substantially from its use elsewhere in medieval literature: typically, leprosy is a chastisement ordered by God, not a condition imitated by a man for the purpose of concealing his identity. Nonetheless, whether the leprosy is a disguise or divine punishment, it always has moral significance. In *Frauendienst,* the Tristan legend, *Jaufré,* and *The Testament of Cresseid,* the leprosy is linked with physical lust; in *The Testament of Cresseid* and *Der Arme Heinrich* it punishes the sin of pride; and in the Amis and Amiloun story as in Dante, it is the consequence of falsification. In short, the association of leprosy with spiritual defilement is pervasive in the literature of the Middle Ages, and not arbitrarily so, but because common beliefs—as seen in medical, homiletic, and social attitudes —made the same connection.

The association of leprosy with morality does not end

with the waning of the Middle Ages; in fact it continues into the twentieth century. Since a detailed examination of later attitudes is beyond the scope of this book, I will conclude with a brief account.

Medical histories generally agree that during the sixteenth century leprosy ceased to be prevalent in Europe and became limited to certain isolated areas. Nevertheless, the disease remained a powerful literary image, suggesting that even if audiences were not familiar with leprosy and had no direct experience with it, the medieval idea of the disease stayed alive. The *Oxford English Dictionary* provides a record of the continuing idea of leprosy as a moral condition. In 1552, a preacher tells his congregation, "so are we lepers of our soules"; a work printed in 1588 also mentions "ye lepre . . . of ye saull"; one writer in 1598 characterizes the time as a "sinne leapered age," and another writes, "My leprosie is a defiled soule." In 1602, John Marston describes a character in a play as "leapred with so foule a guilt"; an entry for 1623 refers to "this leprosie of Atheistical contempt"; one for 1632 mentions "the leprous humour of Popery"; in 1651, Thomas Hobbes writes of men who are "cleansed of the Leprosie of Sin by Faith"; a writer in 1697 confesses to having a "leprous soul"; in 1709 there is mention of those who are "Leprosy'd with Scandal"; in 1751 another entry names the "leprosy of false knowledge"; and in 1781, William Cowper writes the following couplet:

> When nations are to perish in their sins,
> 'Tis in the church the leprosy begins.

The nineteenth century continues the tradition: in 1825, "afraid to join the society of the pious," one man looks upon himself "as a leper"; idleness is described as "a moral leprosy" in 1836; and in 1847 Tennyson writes the lines, "A moral leper, I,/To whom none spake."

Writers after the fifteenth century continue to connect leprosy with sinfulness, and lust—being perhaps the most sensational of sins—is encountered in their writing with great frequency. Shakespeare describes leprosy as venereal in *Timon of Athens* (1606–1609), where Timon puns on the word *whore* when he mentions that gold can be used to buy a woman—it will make "the hoar leprosy adored" (IV.iii.35)[46]; and in *Henry V* (1600), Pistol tells Nym to go to the hospital and find the leprous woman named Doll Tearsheet and marry her:

> No, to the spital go,
> And from the powdering tub of infamy
> Fetch forth the lazar kite of Cressid's kind,
> Doll Tearsheet she by name, and her espouse.
> [II.i.78–81]

In the play *'Tis Pity She's a Whore* (before 1633), by John Ford,[47] there is a brother who would love his sister incestuously. A friar counsels him to put his love aside, saying:

> Beg Heaven to cleanse the leprosy of lust
> That rots thy soul. [I.i.74–75]

The brother does not cleanse his leprous soul, however, and his sister is soon pregnant by him. When her fiancé discovers that she is pregnant, he threatens to do harm to

---

[46] Citations from Shakespeare are from *The Complete Works*, ed. G. B. Harrison (New York, 1952). For the same pun on *hoar*, see *Romeo and Juliet*, II.iv.138 ff.

[47] Ed. Brian Morris, A Mermaid Dramabook (New York, 1968).

her "lust-be-lepered body" (IV.iii.60). Such references to leprosy in drama confirm that the tie between leprosy and sexuality was current not only among educated persons, but also in the popular culture generally, and the idea remained so well after the Middle Ages had ended.

For example, an article in the medical journal *The Lancet*, in the volume for 1823–1824, prints a description of leprosy in India written by an indigo planter.[48] The writer observes that lepers have "no excessive propensity to venery after the disease appears, although they may have had it before." In a desire to correct what he calls "common opinion," he emphasizes that lepers are not "of a warm and amourous temperament." Common opinion is, if nothing else, pervasive, and the common opinion that leprosy is the consequence of lust was voiced with regularity during the nineteenth century. A textbook on leprosy published in 1901 discredits any great role that sexual intercourse might have as a mode of infection, but its remarks on popular attitudes reveal the persistence of the theory. The venereal mode of infection is said to be generally accepted by the laity and also by many physicians as the primary way of spreading the disease. Two Hawaiian patients are reported to have stated "that their principal dread of having the real nature of the disease known was that it would carry to the minds of their friends a conviction of their immorality."[49] Their fear was well founded, as the famous

[48] "Description of the Indian Leprosy," *The Lancet*, II (1823–1824), 149–150.

[49] Prince A. Morrow, "Leprosy," in *Twentieth Century Practice: An International Encyclopedia of Modern Medical Science*, ed. Thomas L. Stedman, XVIII (New York, 1901), 448 f. Cf. Zachary Gussow and George S. Tracy, "Stigma and the Leprosy Phenomenon: The Social History of a Disease in the Nineteenth

case of Father Damien proves. Father Damien, who worked at the leprosarium in Molokai, Hawaii, contracted leprosy and died of it after about fifteen years, in 1889. Three months after his death, the Rev. Charles McEwen Hyde, head of the Presbyterian mission in Honolulu, explained in a letter how the priest became a leper: "He was not a pure man in his relations with women, and the leprosy of which he died should be attributed to his vices and carelessness."[50] The accusation easily gained currency, for people were prepared to accept the logic that if the priest became a leper, then he must have had sexual intercourse with lepers.

In the ninetenth century, a general misapprehension of leprosy, and in particular of leprosy as a venereal disease, was still to be expected. The differential diagnosis of leprosy could be made only after careful studies in the middle of the century had led to reasonably complete and accurate descriptions of the disease, and the impact of those studies was only slowly felt, even in the medical community. Additionally, certain social and political developments during the century worked to reinforce some of the old ideas about leprosy. Western colonialism brought colonists into Asia, Africa, and the subcontinent of India, where leprosy is endemic. The outbreak of leprosy in Hawaii in the 1860's caused fear that the disease might spread among the colonies generally and ultimately among Western nations. At the same time, the work of bacteriologists and

---

and Twentieth Centuries," *Bull Hist Med*, XLIV (1970), 442–443, who quote a report (1893) that Hawaiians possessed "absolute fearlessness and absence of disgust for the disease."

[50] Quoted in Patrick Feeny, *The Fight against Leprosy* (London, 1964), pp. 88–89.

pharmacologists was suggesting that leprosy, a highly contagious disease, was also incurable. The Western response to leprosy was thus highly charged, and not least of all because the disease was found among people believed to be racially inferior to Westerners. Because colonial nations met the leprosy threat by segregating lepers in the colonies and limiting the immigration of selected foreign populations, colonial missionaries were essentially alone in caring for lepers, and the missionaries (who could provide little in the way of medical care) took their responsibility to be the care of the souls of lepers. "Thus, leprosy began, more and more, to be thought of less as a disease than as a moral condition, or as a disease with a moral diagnosis."[51] In short, with the renewed threat of leprosy in the last decades of the nineteenth century, there was also a renewal of old ideas of leprosy, including traditional Christian attitudes.

The nineteenth century's inaccurate and morally charged picture of leprosy was carried over into the twentieth century. The *Oxford English Dictionary* (1933), ordinarily characterized by objectivity and precision, lacks both in its definition of leprosy. Whereas it defines syphilis clinically—"a specific disease caused by *Treponema pallidum* (*Spirochaete pallida*) and communicated by sexual connexion or accidental contact (acquired form) or by infection of the child in utero (congenital form)"—the definition of leprosy conveys moral and aesthetic distaste and mistaken medical information: "a loathsome disease (*Elephantiasis Graecorum*), which slowly eats away the body, and forms shining white scales on the skin." Leprosy lesions are never white, except when there is scarring; the

[51] Gussow and Tracy, pp. 425–449.

white scales are not the result of empirical reporting but can be traced ultimately back to the Bible (in II Kings 5:27, Gehazi is described as "a leper as white as snow"; Leviticus 13:10 identifies "a white color in the skin" as a sign of leprosy) and to the Greek word *lepos*, "a scale," which is the etymological source of Greek *lepra*, "leprosy."

A book on leprosy by Paolo Zappa, *Unclean! Unclean!*, published in London in the same year as the *Oxford English Dictionary*, also illustrates the persistence of conventional misapprehensions of leprosy. The author writes that "it is a very short step between leprosy and madness"; he reports that out of a "Satanic feeling" lepers spread their disease sadistically in order to gain comfort from seeing others suffer with them; and he finds from conversations with lepers both that the disease is spread through sexual intercourse and that it heightens sexual desire. Zappa provides an account, drawn from a leper's diary, of the progress of the disease. The diary tells how the unfortunate man spent some time on an island in the South Pacific, and how one night in June, after a "throbbing, sensual orgy," he had sexual intercourse on the beach with one of the native women. By late August, the diarist writes of a growing sense of evil within him, and the first signs of leprosy arrive with the beginning of September. By January, an entry reads, "Extraordinary! The inner decomposition gives me the strangest, most voluptuous sensations." Within a month, the fingers of the leper's hand snap off "like a dry twig."[52]

The fingers of lepers' hands do not snap off, however. The writer is merely repeating one of the common myths

[52] Paolo Zappa, *Unclean! Unclean!*, trans. Edward Storer (London, 1933), pp. 93, 136, 97–98, 118–129.

about leprosy. James A. Michener, who ought to know better, also uses the myth in his novel *Hawaii*. He describes lepers "whose lips and noses had fallen away," or whose "feet had fallen away," or whose lips "were about to fall away," leaving the impression that the loss of lips, noses, and feet is something other than a gradual process. "Her shattered husband had already begun to lose his toes and fingers." In addition, although Michener does not explicitly state that lepers are excessively sexual, he describes the fate of "an uncommonly pretty girl" whose beauty "excites" three lepers: she is raped by them, kept by them for their own pleasure for five days, enjoyed by more than eighteen men for six weeks, and then "turned loose for whoever wanted her." Michener tells us that this sort of thing was common practice among the male lepers, even those in advanced stages of the disease. And he does not exempt the women. Together with the men they brew liquor, stay drunk for weeks at a time, and wind up "in some public place, naked and lustful, there to indulge themselves with one another to the applause of cheering witnesses."[53]

These descriptions of the immorality of lepers are obviously in a tradition which goes back to the Middle Ages. It is striking that each of the observations made by Paolo Zappa about lepers duplicates the writings of medieval authors. Zappa states that the disease is venereal, and this belief is found everywhere in medieval culture. Zappa writes of the voluptuousness, of the "strange unbridled desire" encountered among lepers, and his writing echoes Aretaeus' report of the lepers' "irresistable and shameless

[53] James A. Michener, *Hawaii* (New York, 1959), pp. 487–496.

impulse for intercourse." In the same way, Zappa's comments on the lepers' "sense of evil" and "sadistic desire to increase the number of companions in misery" recall Edward III's warning that lepers infect others so that "to their own wretched solace, they may have the more fellows in suffering."

The stigma that Zappa attaches to leprosy is clearly the stigma attached to it in medieval culture. The moral implications of the disease were so firmly established in Western culture during the medieval period that they have lasted into our own time. A survey of medieval attitudes toward leprosy shows that the society took over ideas received from classical antiquity, elaborated them, and circulated them so that they infused all aspects of the culture, whether religious, medical, legal, literary, or popular. The stigma of leprosy is thus the product of a long tradition, and that tradition has survived because it is the expression of a complex array of cultural forces.

Works Cited

Texts

Adamus Scotus. *Sermones*. PL, CXCVIII.

Aelfric. *The Homilies of The Anglo-Saxon Church: The First Part, Containing the Sermones Catholici, or Homilies of Aelfric*. Ed. and trans. Benjamin Thorpe. 2 vols. London: The Aelfric Society, 1844–1846.

Alain de Lille. *Liber in distinctionibus dictionum theologicalium*. PL, CCX.

Altdeutsche Predigten. Ed. Anton E. Schönbach. 3 vols. Graz: Verlags-Buchhandlung Styria, 1886–1891.

Amis and Amiloun. *Amis and Amiloun*. Ed. MacEdward Leach. EETS, O.S., no. 203. London: Oxford Univ. Press, 1937.

———. *Amis and Amiloun zugleich mit der altfranzösischen quelle*. Ed. Eugen Kölbing. Altenglische Bibliothek, Vol. II. Heilbronn: Henninger, 1844.

———. *Amis et Amile. Nouvelles Françoises en Prose du XIIIe Siècle*. Ed. L. Moland and C. D'Héricault. Paris: Jannet, 1856.

———. *Amis et Amiles und Jourdains de Blaivies*. Ed. Konrad Hofmann. 2d ed. Erlangen: Deichert, 1882.

———. *Miracle de Nostre Dame d'Amis et d'Amille*. Vol. IV of *Miracles de Nostre Dame par Personnages*. Ed. Gaston Paris and Ulysse Robert. SATF. Paris, 1879.

Ancrene Wisse: The English Text of the Ancrene Riwle. Ed. J. R. R. Tolkien. EETS, no. 249. London: Oxford University Press, 1962.

Anthony of Padua. *Sancti Francisci Assisiatis . . . nec non S. Antonii Paduani . . . Opera Omnia. . . .* Ed. Joannes de la Haye. Stadt am Hof: sumptibus Joannis Gastl, 1739.

Aretaeus. *The Extant Works of Aretaeus, the Cappadocian.* Ed. and trans. Francis Adams. London: Sydenham Society, 1856.

Articuli observandi inter Fratres professos Domus Sancti Juliani, juxta Sanctum Albanum. "Appendix C." *Gesta Abbatum Sancti Albani.* Ed. Henry Thomas Riley. Vol. II. London: Longmans, Green, Reader, and Dyer, 1867.

Bartholomeus Anglicus. *De Proprietatibus Rerum.* Trans. John Trevisa. London: in aedibus Thomae Bertheleti, 1535.

Bede. *In Pentateuchum Commentarii. PL,* XCI.

Béroul. *The Romance of Tristran by Beroul: A Poem of the Twelfth Century.* Ed. A. Ewert. Oxford: Blackwell, 1939.

Bersuire, Pierre. *Opera omnia totam S. Scripturae. . . .* 3 vols. in 2. Antwerp: apud Ioannem Keerbergivm, 1609.

Bible. *Bibliorum Sacrorum iuxta Vulgatam Clementinam.* Ed. Alosius Gramatica. 2d ed. Rome: Vatican Press, 1959.

——. *The Holy Bible: Translated from the Latin Vulgate.* Baltimore: Murphy, 1914.

——. *Proverbs, Ecclesiastes.* Trans. R. B. Y. Scott. The Anchor Bible, vol. XVIII. Garden City, N.Y.: Doubleday, 1965.

——. *The Torah: The Five Books of Moses.* Trans. Harry M. Orlinsky et al. Philadelphia: The Jewish Publication Society of America, 1962.

——. *II Chronicles.* Trans. Jacob M. Myers. The Anchor Bible, vol. XIII. Garden City, N.Y.: Doubleday, 1965.

Bodel, Jean. "Les Congés de Jean Bodel." Ed. Gaston Raynaud. *Romania,* IX (1880), 216–247.

The Book of Vices and Virtues: A Fourteenth Century English Translation of the "Somme le Roi" of Lorens d'Orleans. Ed. W. Nelson Francis. EETS, O.S., no. 217. London: Oxford Univ. Press, 1942.

Bracton, Henry de. *Bracton's Note Book: A Collection of Cases Decided in the King's Courts during the Reign of Henry the Third.* Ed. F. W. Maitland. 3 vols. London: Clay, 1887.

——. *Henrici de Bracton De legibus & consuetudinibus Angliae.* London: apud Richardum Totellum, 1569.

Brown, M. Webster. "Two Ancient Descriptions of Lepers." *Med J Rec,* CXXXVII (1933), 299.

Caesarius of Arles. *Sermones.* Ed. Germanus Morin. 1 vol. in 2 pts. Maretioli, 1937.

——, *Sermons.* Trans. Sister Mary Magdeleine Mueller, 2 vols. The Fathers of the Church, vols. XXXI, XLVII. New York: Fathers of the Church, 1956–64.

Caesarius of Heisterbach. *The Dialogue on Miracles.* Trans. H. von E. Scott and C. C. Swinton Bland. 2 vols. London: Routledge, 1929.

Chaucer, Geoffrey. *The Works of Geoffrey Chaucer.* Ed. Fred N. Robinson. 2d ed. Boston: Houghton Mifflin, 1957.

Concilium Vaurense. Sacrorum conciliorum nova et amplissima collectio. Ed. Phil. Labbeus et al. Vol. XXVI. Graz: Akademische Druck- u. Verlagsanstalt, 1961. Pp. 474–547.

Dan Michel's Ayenbite of Inwit. Ed. Richard Morris. EETS, no. 23. London: Trübner, 1866.

Dante Alighieri. *The Divine Comedy of Dante Alighieri.* Trans. John D. Sinclair. 3 vols. New York: Oxford Univ. Press, 1948.

De antiquis Ecclesiae ritibus libri ex variis insigniorum Eccelsiarum . . . Ed. Edmund Martène. 4 vols. Antwerp: de la Bry, 1736–1738.

"Description of the Indian Leprosy." *The Lancet,* II (1823–1824), 149–150.

Eilhart von Oberge. *Tristram und Isolde. Eilhart von Oberge.* Ed. Franz Lichtenstein. *QFSK,* vol. XIX. Strassburg: Trübner, 1877.

English Metrical Homilies: From Manuscripts of the Four-teenth Century. Ed. John Small. Edinburgh: Paterson, 1862.

Fastoul, Baude. "Che sont li Congié Baude Fastoul d'Aras." *Fabliaux et contes des poètes françois.* Ed. Étienne Barbazan and M. Méon. 4 vols. Paris: Warée, 1808.

Ford, John. *'Tis Pity She's a Whore.* Ed. Brian Morris. A Mermaid Dramabook. New York: Hill and Wang, 1968.

Fracastorius, Hieronymous. *De contagione et contagiosis morbis et eorum curatione, libri III.* Ed. and trans. Wilmer Cave Wright. New York: Putnam's Sons, 1930.

Garner of Rochefort. *Allegoriae in Sacram Scripturam.* PL, CXII. Attributed by Migne to Hrabanus Maurus.

Gauthier de Châtillon. *Die Gedichte Walters von Chatillon.* Ed. Karl Strecker. Berlin: Weidmann, 1925.

Gesta Romanorum. *The Early English Version of the Gesta Romanorum.* Ed. Sidney J. H. Herrtage. EETS, E.S., no. 33. London: Trübner, 1879.

——. *Die Gesta Romanorum.* Ed. Wilhelm Dick. *Erlanger Beiträge zur Englischen Philologie,* VII (1890), 1–273.

——. *Gesta Romanorum: Entertaining Moral Stories.* Trans. Charles Swan. London: Routledge; New York: Dutton, 1905.

Ginzberg, Louis. *The Legends of the Jews.* Trans. Henrietta Szold and Paul Radin. 7 vols. Philadelphia: Jewish Publication Society of America, 1909–1938.

Glossa Ordinaria. PL, CXIII.

Gower, John. *Confessio Amantis. The Complete Works of John Gower.* Ed. G. C. Macaulay. 4 vols. Oxford: Clarendon Press, 1899–1902.

Graves, Robert, and Raphael Patai. *Hebrew Myths: The Book of Genesis.* New York: Doubleday, 1964.

Gregorius IX. *Decretales.* Basel: Froben, 1494.

Gregory the Great. *Moralium libri.* PL, LXXV–LXXXVI.

——. *Morals on the Book of Job.* A Library of the Fathers of the Holy Catholic Church, vols. XVIII, XXI, XXIII, XXXI. Oxford: Library of the Fathers, 1844–1850.

Gregory of Nazianzus. "Oratio XLIII: In laudem Basilii Magni." *PG*, XXXVI.

Gregory of Nysse. *De pauperibus amandis, oratio II. PG*, XLVI.

Guy of Chauliac. *La Grande Chirvrgie.* Ed. E. Nicaise. Paris: Alcan, 1890.

——. *The questyonary of Cyrurgyens, with the formulary of lytell Guydo in Cyrurgie . . . newly Enprynted at London, by me Robert Wyer.* Trans. Robert Copland. London, 1542.

Hartman von Aue. *Der Arme Heinrich.* Ed. Erich Gierach and J. Knight Bostock. 4th ed. Oxford: Blackwell, 1965.

Henryson, Robert. *The Poems and Fables of Robert Henryson.* Ed. H. Harvey Wood. 2d ed. Edinburgh: Oliver and Boyd, 1958.

——. *Testament of Cresseid.* Ed. Denton Fox. First published London: Nelson and Sons, 1968; Old & Middle English Texts, Manchester: Manchester University Press, 1968.

Hermann von Fritzlar. "Sanct Silvester: Tischrede aus dem Buch von der Heiligen Leben." *Der Arme Heinrich Herrn Hartmanns von Aue und Zwei Jüngere Prosalegenden verwandten Inhaltes.* Ed. Wilhelm Wackernagel and Ernst Stadler. Basel: Schwabe, 1911.

Hrabanus Maurus. *Allegoriae in Sacram Scripturam.* See Garner of Rochefort.

——. *De universo. PL*, CXI.

Hugh of St. Victor. *Allegoriae.* See Richard of St. Victor.

Isidore of Seville. *Allegoriae quaedam Sacrae Scripturae. PL*, LXXXIII.

——. *Quaestiones in Vetus Testamentum. PL*, LXXXIII.

Jacques de Vitry. *The Exempla or Illustrative Stories from the Sermones Vulgares of Jacques de Vitry.* Ed. Thomas Frederick Crane. Publications of the Folk-Lore Society, vol. XXVI. London: Nutt, 1890.

Jaufré: Roman arthurien du XIIIe siècle en vers provençaux. Ed. Clovis Brunel. SATF. 2 vols. Paris, 1943.

Jerome, Saint. *Allegoriae in Novum Testamentum.* PL, CLXXV.

——. *Scripta supposititia: Epistolae.* PL, XXX.

Joannes Cassianus. *De coenobiorum institutis.* PL, XLIX.

Joinville, Jean, Sire de. *Histoire de Saint Louis, Credo, et Lettre à Louis X.* Ed. and trans. Natalis de Wailly. 2d ed. Paris: Didot frères, fils et Cie., 1874.

Justin Martyr. *The Writings of Justin Martyr and Athenagoras.* Trans. Marcus Dods, George Reith, and B. P. Pratten. The Ante-Nicene Christian Library, vol. II. Edinburg: Clark, 1870.

A Leechbook or Collection of Medical Recipes of the Fifteenth Century. Ed. and trans. Warren R. Dawson. London: Macmillan, 1934.

Lydgate, John. *Lydgate's Fall of Princes.* Ed. Henry Bergen. Carnegie Institute of Washington, no. 262. 4 vols. Washington: Carnegie Institute of Washington, 1923–1927.

Maimonides, Moses. *The Guide for the Perplexed.* Trans. M. Friedländer. 4th ed. New York: Dutton, 1927.

Mannyng, Robert, of Brunne. *Robert of Brunne's "Handlyng Synne," A.D. 1303, with Those Parts of the Anglo-French Treatise on which It was Founded, William of Wadington's "Manuel des Pechiez."* Ed. Frederick J. Furnivall. EETS, O.S., nos. 119, 123. London: Paul, Trench, Trübner, 1901–1903.

Maurice of Sully. *Maurice of Sully and the Medieval Vernacular Homily: with the Text of Maurice's French Homilies from a Sens Cathedral Chapter MS.* Ed. C. A. Robson. Oxford: Blackwell, 1952.

Memorials of London and London Life. Ed. and trans. Henry Thomas Riley. London: London Corporation, 1868.

Michener, James A. *Hawaii.* New York: Random House, 1959.

Middle English Sermons. Ed. Woodburn O. Ross. EETS, O.S., no. 209. London: Oxford Univ. Press, 1940.

Midrash Rabbah. Ed. H. Freedman and Maurice Simon. 10 vols. London: Soncino Press, 1939.

Migne, J. P., ed. *Patrologiae cursus completus: Series graeca.* 162 vols. Paris: Migne, 1857–1866.

——. *Patrologiae cursus completus: Series latina.* 221 vols. in 222. Paris: Garnier fratres, 1844–1880.

Mikra'oth Gedoloth. 5 vols. New York: Tanach, 1959.

Morrow, Prince A. "Leprosy." *Twentieth Century Practice: An International Encyclopedia of Modern Medical Science.* Ed. Thomas L. Stedman. New York: Wood, 1901. XVIII, 403–683.

An Old English Miscellany. Ed. Richard Morris. EETS, O.S., no. 49. London: Trübner, 1872.

Prudentius. *Prudentius.* Ed. and trans. H. J. Thomson. The Loeb Classical Library. 2 vols. Cambridge, Mass.: Harvard Univ. Press, 1949–1953.

Radulphus Flaviacensis. *Commentatiorum in Leuiticum Libri XX.* Ed. Margarino de la Bigne. Maxima Bibliotheca Vetervm Patrvm, et Antiqvorvm Scriptorvm Ecclesiasticorvm, vol. XVII. London: apud Anissonios, 1677.

Registrum omnium breuium tam originalium quam iudicialium. London: William Rastell, 1531.

Richard of St. Victor. *Allegoriae in Novum Testamentum.* PL, CLXXV. Attributed by Migne to Hugh of St. Victor.

——. *Allegoriae in Vetus Testamentum.* PL, CLXXV. Attributed by Migne to Hugh of St. Victor.

Rupert of Deutz. *De trinitate et operibus ejus.* PL, CLXVII.

Rutebeuf. "La Disputaison de Charlot et du Barbier." *Oeuvres complètes de Rutebeuf.* Ed. Edmond Faral and Julia Bastin. 2 vols. Paris: Picard, 1959–1960.

Shakespeare, William. *The Complete Works.* Ed. G. B. Harrison. New York: Harcourt, Brace and World, 1952.

Statuts d'hôtels-dieu et de léproseries: Recueil de textes du XIIe au XIVe siècle. Ed. Léon Le Grand. Paris: Picard, 1901.

Tertullian. *Adversus Marcionem Libri Quinque*. PL, II.

——. *De pudicitia*. PL, II.

——. *The Five Books of Quintus Sept. Flor. Tertullianus against Marcion*. Trans. Peter Holmes. The Ante-Nicene Christian Library, vol. III. Edinburgh: Clark, 1870.

——. *Treatises on Penance: On Penitence and On Purity*. Trans. William P. Le Saint. Ancient Christian Writers, no. 28. Westminster, Maryland: Newman Press, 1959.

Theodoric of Cervia. *The Surgery of Theodoric*. Trans. Eldridge Campbell and James Colton. 2 vols. New York: Appleton-Century-Crofts, 1955–1960.

"A Thirteenth Century Clinical Description of Leprosy." Ed. and trans. Charles Singer. *J Hist Med*, IV (1949), 237–239.

Thomas. *Gottfried von Strassburg, Tristan . . . with the surviving fragments of the Tristran of Thomas*. Trans. A. T. Hatto. Baltimore: Penguin Books, 1960.

——. *Le Roman de Tristan par Thomas*. Ed. Joseph Bédier. SATF. 2 vols. Paris, 1902–1905.

"Two Ancient Descriptions of Lepers." Trans. M. Webster Brown. *Med J Rec*, CXXXVII (1933), 299.

Ulrich von Lichtenstein. *Ulrich's von Liechtenstein Frauendienst*. Ed. Reinhold Bechstein. 2 vols. Leipzig: Brockhaus, 1888.

Wistasse le Moine: Altfranzösischer Abenteuerroman des XIII. Jahrhunderts. Ed. Wendelin Foerster and Johann Trost. Halle: Niemeyer, 1891.

Wyclif, John. *The English Works of Wyclif Hitherto Unprinted*. Ed. F. D. Matthew. EETS, O.S., no. 74. London: Trübner, 1880.

Secondary Sources

Adams, Francis, ed. and trans. *The Seven Books of Paulus Aegineta*. 3 vols. London: Sydenham Society, 1844–1847.

Aiken, Pauline. "The Summoner's Malady." *SP*, XXXIII (1936), 40–44.

Amato, Vincenzo d'. *La Lebbre nella Storia, nella Geografia e nell' Arte*. Rome: Stabilimento Tipografico Romano, 1923.

Ball, C. J., ed. and trans. *The Book of Job*. Oxford: Clarendon Press, 1922.

Bauer, Walter. *A Greek-English Lexicon of The New Testament and other Early Christian Literature*. Trans. William F. Arndt and F. Wilbur Gingrich. 4th ed. Chicago: Univ. of Chicago Press, 1957.

Binford, Chapman H. "Leprosy." *Communicable and Infectious Diseases*. Ed. Franklin H. Top. 4th ed. St. Louis: Mosby, 1960.

Blaise, Albert. *Dictionnaire Latin-Française des auteurs Chrétiens*. Turnhout, Beligium: Éditions Brepols, 1954.

Bloomfield, Morton W. *The Seven Deadly Sins*. East Lansing: Michigan State Univ. Press, 1952.

Boas, George. *Essays on Primitivism and Related Ideas in the Middle Ages*. New York: Octagon Books, 1966.

Bowden, Muriel. *A Commentary on the General Prologue to The Canterbury Tales*. New York: Macmillan, 1948.

Calin, William. *The Epic Quest: Studies in Four Old French Chansons de Geste*. Baltimore: The Johns Hopkins Press, 1966.

Carlowitz, [Constantin] Hans, ed. *Der Lepraabschnitt aus Bernhard von Gordons "Lillium medicinae" in mittelalterlicher deutscher Uebersetzung*. Leipzig: Peter, 1913.

Cassel, Paulus. *Die Symbolik des Blutes und "Der arme Heinrich" von Hartmann von Aue*. Berlin: Hoffmann, 1882.

Chevalier, J. A. Ulysse. *Notice historique sur la maladrerie de Voley près Romans*. Romans: Rosier, 1870.

Clay, Rotha Mary. *The Medieval Hospitals of England*. London: Methuen, 1909.

Cochrane, R. G., ed. *Leprosy in Theory and Practice*. 1st ed. Bristol: Wright, 1959.

——, and T. Frank Davey, eds., *Leprosy in Theory and Practice*. 2d ed. Bristol: Wright, 1964.

Cougoul, Jacques-Guy. *La Lèpre dans l'Ancienne France*. Bordeaux: Delmas, 1943.

Crosland, Jessie. *The Old French Epic*. Oxford: Blackwell, 1951.

Curry, Walter Clyde. *Chaucer and the Medieval Sciences*. New York: Oxford Univ. Press, 1926.

Curtius, Ernst Robert. *European Literature and the Latin Middle Ages*. Trans. Willard R. Trask. New York: Harper and Row, 1963.

Delaunay, Paul. "Histoire de la Médecine: De la condition des lépreux au Moyen Age." *Hippocrate*, II (1934), 456–460.

Dupouy, Edmond. *Le Moyen Age Médical*. Paris: Société d'Éditions Scientifiques, 1895.

Eggtling, H. Julius. "Sanskrit." *Encyclopaedia Britannica*. 11th ed. XXIV, 156–183.

Expert Committee on Leprosy: Second Report. World Health Organization Technical Report Series, no. 189. Geneva, 1960.

Fechter, Werner, "Uber den 'Armen Heinrich' Hartmanns von Aue." *Euphorion*, XLIX (1955), 1–28.

Feeny, Patrick. *The Fight against Leprosy*. London: Elek Books, 1964.

Ferguson, George. *Signs and Symbols in Christian Art*. New York: Oxford Univ. Press, 1961.

Fite, George L. "Book Review: *Leprosy in Theory and Practice*." *Int J Leprosy*, XXVII (1959), 300–302.

Fletcher, Angus. *Allegory: The Theory of a Symbolic Mode*. Ithaca, N.Y.: Cornell Univ. Press, 1964.

Foulon, Charles. *L'Oeuvre de Jehan Bodel*. Rennes: Imprimeries Réunis, 1958.

Gombrich, E. H. *Art and Illusion: A Study in the Psychology of Pictorial Representation*. New York: Pantheon Books, 1960.

Gussow, Zachery and George S. Tracy. "Stigma and the Leprosy Phenomenon: The Social History of a Disease in the Nineteenth and Twentieth Centuries." *Bull Hist Med*, XLIV (1970), 425–449.

Haggard, Howard W. *Devils, Drugs, and Doctors*. New York: Harper and Bros., 1929.

Harmand, Auguste. *Notice historique sur la léproserie de la ville de Troyes*. Mémoires de la Société d'Agriculture, des Sciences, Arts et Belles-Lettres du Département de l'Aube. 2d series, vol. I, nos. 7–8. Troyes, 1848.

Harth, Sydney. "Henryson Reinterpreted." *EIC*, XI (1961), 471–480.

Hartley, Percival Horton-Smith and Harold Richard Aldridge. *Johannes de Mirfeld of St. Bartholomew's, Smithfield: His Life and Works*. Cambridge, England: The University Press, 1936.

Hildenfinger, Paul. *La Léproserie de Reims du XIIe au XVIIe siècle*. Reims: Michaud, 1906.

Holcomb, R[ichmond] C. "The Antiquity of Congenital Syphilis." *Bull Hist Med*, X (1941), 148–177.

——. *Who Gave the World Syphilis?* New York: Froben Press, 1937.

Holdsworth, W. S. *A History of English Law*. 3d ed. 9 vols. Boston: Methuen, 1922–1924.

Holländer, Eugen. *Die Medezin in der klassischen Malerei*. 3d ed. Stuttgart: Enke, 1923.

Huber, Raphael M. *St. Anthony of Padua, Doctor of the Church Universal*. Milwaukee: Bruce, 1948.

Huizinga, Lee S. "Leprosy in Legend and History: King Bladud of England." *Leper Quart*, XIII (1939), 18–20.

Indice Bibliografico de Lepra. Ed. Luiza Keffer. 3 vols. São Paulo: Departamento de Profilaxia da Lepra, 1944–1948.

Innes, J. Ross. "An Approach to the History of Leprosy." *Ciba Symposium*, VII (1959), 117–123.

The Interpreter's Bible. Ed. George Arthur Buttrick et al. 12 vols. New York: Abington-Cokesbury, 1951–1957.

Jeanselme, E. "Comment l'Europe, au Moyen Age, se protégea contre la lèpre." *Bull Soc fr Hist Med,* XXV (1931), 1–155.

Jonin, Pierre. *Les Personnages féminins dans les romans français de Tristan au XIIe siècle: Étude des influences contemporaines.* Publication des annales de la faculté des lettres, Aix-en-Provence. New series, no. 22. Gap: Ophrys, 1958.

Kaufmann, Yehezkel. *The Religion of Israel: From Its Beginnings to the Babylonian Exile.* Trans. Moshe Greenberg. Chicago: Univ. of Chicago Press, 1960.

Kratins, Ojars. "The Middle English *Amis and Amiloun:* Chivalric Romance or Secular Hagiography?" *PMLA,* LXXXI (1966), 347–354.

Langlade, Emile. *Jehan Bodel: Avec des commentaires sur le Congé de Baude Fastoul.* Paris: Rudeval, 1909.

Lubac, Henri de. *Exégèse médiévale: Les quatre sens de l'Écriture.* 2 vols. Paris: Aubier, 1959–1964.

Macalister, Alexander. "Leprosy." *A Dictionary of the Bible.* Ed. James Hastings et al. Vol. III. New York: Scribner's, 1901.

MacArthur, William, "Medieval 'Leprosy' in the British Isles." *Leprosy Rev,* XXIV (1953), 8–19.

——. "Some Notes on Old-Time Leprosy in England and Ireland." *J Roy Army Med Corps,* XLV (1925), 410–422.

MacKinney, Loren C. *Early Medieval Medicine: With Special Reference to France and Chartres.* Baltimore: The Johns Hopkins Press, 1937.

Maury, Alfred. *Croyances et légendes du Moyen Age.* Paris: Champion, 1896.

Mercier, Charles A. *Leper Houses and Mediaeval Hospitals.* London: Lewis, 1915.

Mettler, Cecelia C. *History of Medicine.* Ed. Fred A. Mettler. Philadelphia: Blakiston, 1947.

Muir, Ernest. *Manual of Leprosy*. Baltimore: Williams and Wilkins, 1948.

Nagel, Bert. *Der Arme Heinrich Hartmanns von Aue. Eine Interpretation*. Tübingen: Niemeyer, 1952.

Nemetz, Anthony. "Literalness and the *Sensus Litteralis*." *Spec*, XXXIV (1959), 76–89.

Newman, George. "On the History of the Decline and Final Extinction of Leprosy as an Endemic Disease in the British Islands." *Prize Essays on Leprosy*. The New Sydenham Society, vol. CLVII. London: The New Sydenham Society, 1895.

Obermann, Julian, ed. *The Code of Maimonides: Book Ten, The Book of Cleanness*. Trans. Herbert Danby. Yale Judaica Series, vol. VIII. New Haven: Yale Univ. Press, 1954.

Owst, G. R. *Preaching in Medieval England: An Introduction to Sermon Manuscripts of the Period c. 1350–1450*. Cambridge, Eng.: University Press, 1926.

Parr, Johnstone. "Cresseid's Leprosy Again." *MLN*, LX (1945), 487–491.

Pollock, Frederick, and Frederic William Maitland. *The History of English Law before the Time of Edward I*. 2d ed. 2 vols. Cambridge, Eng.: University Press; Boston: Little, Brown, 1899.

Remy, Paul. "La lèpre, thème littéraire au moyen âge: Commentaire d'un passage du roman provençal de Jaufré." *MA*, LII (1946), 195–242.

"Research Barrier Breached: Leprosy Bacillus Grown in Tissue Culture." *JAMA*, CXCII, no. 12 (1965), 32–33.

Riesman, David. *The Story of Medicine in the Middle Ages*. New York: Hoeber, 1935.

Roueché, Berton. "A Lonely Road." *Eleven Blue Men: And Other Narratives of Medical Detection*. New York: Berkley, 1953.

Rowland, Beryl. "The 'seiknes incurabill' in Henryson's *Testament of Cresseid*." *ELN*, I (1963–1964), 175–177.

212   *Works Cited*

Schiller, Gertrud. *Ikonographie der christlichen Kunst.* 2 vols. Gütersloh: Gütersloher Verlagshaus G. Mohn, 1966–1968.

Schirokauer, Arno. "Zur Interpretation des Armen Heinrich." *ZDA,* LXXXIII (1951–1952), 59–78.

Scientific Meeting on Rehabilitation in Leprosy, Vellore, Madras State, India, 21–29 November, 1960: Report. World Health Organization Technical Report Series, no. 221. Geneva: World Health Organization, 1961.

Sieffert, Leslie. "The Maiden's Heart: Legend and Fairy-Tale in Hartmann's 'Der Arme Heinrich,' " *DVLG,* XXXVII (1963), 384–405.

Sigerist, Henry E. "Bedside Manners in the Middle Ages: The Treatise *De Cautelis Medicorum* Attributed to Arnald of Villanova." *Henry E. Sigerist on the History of Medicine.* Ed. Felix Marti-Ibañez. New York: MD Publications, 1960.

Simpson, J. Y. "Antiquarian Notices of Leprosy and Leper Hospitals in Scotland and England." *Edin Med Surg J,* LVI (1841), 301–330; LVII (1842), 121–156, 394–429.

Skinsnes, Olaf K. "Leprosy in Society: 'Leprosy Has Appeared on the Face.' " *Leprosy Rev,* XXXV (1964), 21–35.

Smalley, Beryl. *The Study of the Bible in the Middle Ages.* 2d ed. Oxford: Blackwell, 1952.

Smith, Munroe. *The Development of English Law.* New York: Columbia Univ. Press, 1928.

Spicq, C[eslaus]. *Esquisse d'une histoire de l'exégèse latine au moyen âge.* Bibliothèque Thomiste, vol. XXVI. Paris: Vrin, 1944.

Stearns, Marshall W. *Robert Henryson.* New York: Columbia Univ. Press, 1949.

——. "Robert Henryson and the Leper Cresseid." *MLN,* LIX (1944), 265–269.

Surtees, Robert. *The History and Antiquities of the County Palatine of Durham.* 4 vols. London: Nichols and Son, 1816–1840.

Taylor, Henry Osborn. *The Classical Heritage of the Middle Ages.* New York: Harper and Row, 1958.

Thorndike, Lynn. *A History of Magic and Experimental Science.* 8 vols. New York: Macmillan and Columbia Univ. Press, 1923–1958.

Tillyard, E. M. W. "Henryson: *The Testament of Cresseid,* 1470?" *Five Poems: 1470–1870.* London: Chatto and Windus, 1948.

Vaux, Roland de. *Ancient Israel: Its Life and Institutions.* Trans. John McHugh. New York: McGraw-Hill, 1961.

——. *Studies in Old Testament Sacrifice.* Cardiff: University of Wales Press, 1964.

Viollet, Paul. *Droit privé et sources: Histoire du droit civil français.* 2d ed. Paris: Larose & Forcel, 1893.

Virchow, Rud. "Zur Geschichte des Aussatzes und der Spitäler, besonders in Deutschland." *Arch path Anat Physiol,* XVIII (1859), 138–162, 273–329; XIX (1860), 43–93; XX (1861), 166–198, 459–512.

Wackernagel, Wilhelm. "Abhandlung." *Der Arme Heinrich Herrn Hartmanns von Aue und Zwei Jüngere Prosalegenden Verwandten Inhaltes.* Ed. Wilhelm Wackernagel and Ernst Stadler. Basel: Schwabe, 1911.

Whitwell, J. R. *Syphilis in Earlier Days.* London: Lewis, 1940.

Wickersheimer, Ernest, "Les Accusations d'empoisonnement portées pendant la première moitié du XIVe siècle contre les lépreux et les juifs; leurs relations avec les épidémies de peste." *Comptes-rendus du quatrième congrès international d'histoire de la médecine.* Ed. Tricot-Royer and Laignel-Lavastine. Anvers: Imprimerie De Vlijt, 1927.

Willson, H. B. "Symbol and Reality in 'Der Arme Heinrich.' " *MLR,* LIII (1958), 526–536.

Zappa, Paolo. *Unclean! Unclean!* Trans. Edward Storer. London: Dickson, 1933.

Index

Aaron, 48, 113, fig. 8
Abram, 117–118
Absalom, 150
Adams, Francis, 53
Adamus Scotus, 129
Aelfric, 104 n. 95
Aetius of Amida, 53
Aiken, Pauline, 12 n. 3, 49 n. 46
Alain de Lille (Alan of Lille, Alanus de Insulis), 128
Albucasis (Alsaharavius, al-Zahrawi), 53
Aldridge, Harold Richard, 44 nn. 35–36, 45
Almenar, Juan, 54
Alsaharavius, see Albucasis
Amis and Amiloun, story of, 152n, 159–173
  Amiloun in, compared with Heinrich, 172–173
  Christian ethic in, 161–165
  cure of leprosy in, 169–171
  leprosy and bigamy in, 161, 162–163, 164–165, 166
  leprosy and deceit in, 162–169, 171, 173
  romantic and hagiographic versions, 160–161
  summary of, 159–160
Ancrene Wisse, 135 n. 53, 143 n. 67
Andrew of St. Victor, 120n
Anthony of Padua, Saint, 139
Arabic medical writers, 44, 45, 53
Ardericus, 167
Aretaeus of Cappadocia, 53, 181, 196–197

Der Arme Heinrich, see Hartmann von Aue, Der Arme Heinrich
Arnald of Villanova (Arnold of Villanova, Arnaldus Catalonus), 45, 46
Asylums, see Leprosariums
Avicenna (ibn-Sina), 45
Azariah, 113 n. 10, 142

Badger, L. F., 23 n. 4
Ball, C. J., 124 n. 27
Bartholomaeus Anglicus, 50, 55, 119
Bauer, Walter, 113 n. 9
Bede, 126
Berchorius, Petrus, see Bersuire, Pierre
Bernard de Gordon, see Gordon, Bernard
Béroul, see Tristan and Isolde, story of, by Béroul
Bersuire, Pierre (Petrus Berchorius), 136, 143
Bible, 62 n. 2, 73, 107–108
  Genesis, 117
  Leviticus, 48, 61–62, 108–113, 115, 126, 127, 129, 132, 133, 139
  Numbers, 62 n. 5, 109 n. 5, 113
  Deuteronomy, 62 n. 2, 114, 124 n. 27
  I Samuel (I Kings), 116
  II Samuel (II Kings), 150
  II Kings (IV Kings), 73, 113 n. 10, 114, 128, 133, 195
  II Chronicles, 113 n. 10, 114 n. 11
  Proverbs, 115, 167n

The Disease of the Soul

Designed by R. E. Rosenbaum.
Composed by York Composition Co., Inc.,
in 11 point linotype Janson, 3 points leaded,
with display lines in Weiss Roman and Italic.
Printed letterpress from type by York Composition Co., Inc.,
on Warren's Olde Style India, 60 pound basis,
with the Cornell University Press watermark.
Bound by Vail-Ballou Press
in Columbia book cloth
and stamped in All Purpose foil.